Extending Access to Health Care
through Public-Private Partnerships

The PROSALUD Experience

Other Books by Management Sciences for Health

Beyond the Clinic Walls: Case Studies in Community-Based Distribution
ed. James A. Wolff et al. (W. Hartford, CT: Kumarian Press)

CORE—Cost and Revenue Analysis Tool

**The Family Planning Manager's Handbook: Basic Skills and Tools
for Managing Family Planning Programs**
ed. James A. Wolff, Linda J. Suttenfield, and Susanna C. Binzen
(W. Hartford, CT: Kumarian Press)

**Health Financing Reform in Kenya:
The Fall and Rise of Cost Sharing, 1989–94**
by David Collins et al.

**Lessons from MSH: Strategic Planning:
Reflections on Process and Practice**
by Sylvia Vriesendorp

**Management Strategies for Improving Family Planning Services:
The Family Planning Manager Compendium**
ed. Janice Miller and James A. Wolff

**Managing Drug Supply: The Selection, Procurement, Distribution,
and Use of Pharmaceuticals,** with the World Health Organization
2nd edition (W. Hartford, CT: Kumarian Press)

MOST—Management and Organizational Sustainability Tool

Myths and Realities about the Decentralization of Health Systems
ed. Riitta-Liisa Kolehmainen-Aitken

Private Health Sector Growth in Asia: Issues and Implications
ed. William Newbrander (Chichester, England: John Wiley & Sons)

Stubbs Monograph Series Number 2

Extending Access to Health Care through Public-Private Partnerships

The PROSALUD Experience

Carlos J. Cuéllar
William Newbrander
Gail Price

MSH **MANAGEMENT SCIENCES FOR HEALTH**
Boston

Stubbs Monograph Series
Dr. John Stubbs was a practicing general surgeon and a longtime member of the MSH Board of Directors. He was also a founder of the United Bermuda Party, a frequently elected member of the government of Bermuda, and several times a Minister with various portfolios. An ardent advocate of integration and civil rights, Dr. Stubbs long worked to help make Bermuda an effective example of a multiracial society. Accepting people on their own merits, he was a small-"d" democrat to the core, with colleagues and friends from the least- to the most-advantaged segments of society wherever he went.

Dr. Stubbs studied medicine at McGill University, was a Rhodes Scholar, and was a Sloan Fellow at the Massachusetts Institute of Technology.

The Stubbs Memorial Fund supports the publication of this monograph series on the economics and delivery of health services.

Management Sciences for Health
165 Allandale Rd.
Boston, MA 02130-3400

Tel.: 617-524-7799
Fax: 671-524-2825
E-mail: http://www.msh.org/publications
Orders: bookstore@msh.org

Printed in the United States of America on acid-free paper by Thomson-Shore, Inc. with vegetable oil-based ink.

ISBN 0-913723-63-0

Library of Congress Cataloging-in-Publication Data
Cuéllar, Carlos J., 1954–
    Extending access to health care through public-private partnerships : the PROSALUD experience / Carlos J. Cuéllar, William Newbrander, Gail Price.
        p.   cm. — (Stubbs monograph series ; no. 2)
    Includes bibliographical references and index.
    ISBN 0-913723-63-0 (pbk. : acid-free paper)
    1. Community health services—Bolivia. 2. PROSALUD (Bolivia). 3. Community health services—Developing countries—Finance. I. Newbrander, William C. II. Price, Gail, 1959–   . III. Title. IV. Series.

RA461.C84 2000
362.1'2'0984—dc21   99-052798

⊗ The paper used in this publication meets the minimum requirements of the American National Standard for Information Sciences—Permanence of Paper for Printed Library Materials, ANSI Z39.48-1984.

06   05   04   03   02   01   00   10   9   8   7   6   5   4   3   2   1

*To the staff of PROSALUD,
the communities they serve,
and the government partners
who support their work*

Contents

Foreword

The last decade has confirmed a lesson for health decision-makers that should have been obvious to all of us, but rarely seems to be: that making health services widely available works better when a community organizes itself to use all its resources. PROSALUD, a nonprofit health care organization in Bolivia, was built by the ideas, energy, and vision of many dedicated Bolivian leaders. It has not only changed the way health services are delivered but has also inspired others around the world to look and think beyond established systems for delivering health services.

The search for social justice by many countries has often focused on health. Unfortunately, the widely, often fervently, held belief that everyone should have access to health services as a basic right is usually an example of "the great being the enemy of the good," rhetoric suffocating on reality. The simplistically appealing "health for all" concept has for a generation often seduced political leaders into proclaiming that health care should be, must be, and will be free. With time, however, communities have learned that despite the proclamations, it doesn't happen; health services have costs and there is no free lunch. Rights, to exist in reality, require resources, which are always limited; health care is not exempt from these limitations. The challenge in the real world is to choose, and figure out how to pay for, the most important services. PROSALUD has confirmed that this challenge is manageable and as such is one of the most important health lessons of our time.

This book examines what underlies the great contribution of PRO-SALUD to finding the practical middle ground to improve health: looking at the needs and interests of a community, avoiding the impractical rhetoric of rights, and embracing the political wisdom to bring the strengths of the community, both the public sector and the private sector, together.

—Ronald W. O'Connor, MD
*Chief Executive Officer and Chairman of
the Board, Management Sciences for Health*

Preface

In 1985, against a backdrop of extreme economic difficulties and disheartening health statistics, the Bolivian government was working toward its goal of "health for all by the year 2000." Bolivia had a gross national product of $480 per capita, less than one-third the average of other countries in Latin America. Indicators of health status, such as the mortality rate of children under five of 195 per 1,000, were twice as high as the averages in the region.

In response to these problems, the US Agency for International Development funded a project to provide basic services through an alternative delivery system in the areas surrounding the city of Santa Cruz, Bolivia. Management Sciences for Health signed a cooperative agreement with USAID to provide PROSALUD, a nonprofit Bolivian organization, with technical assistance and financial support. From 1985 to 1990, MSH and PROSALUD worked together to develop a network of self-financing primary health care clinics for low- and middle-income people. Today, these clinics have expanded to cities throughout Bolivia, and they continue to offer affordable, high-quality services, supported by the participation of the community.

Many countries are undergoing health sector reform, the goals of which are to improve access to basic health services and increase their quality while decreasing costs and inefficiencies. As many countries redesign the role of the public sector, public-private collaboration is one of the key strategies being used to effect these changes. Although public-private partnerships are not new to the health sector, they are becoming much more commonplace in many developing countries. Such partnerships involve close collaboration and pooling of resources in a relationship that varies in its degree of formality. Informal relationships between the public and private sectors may have existed for years. These more formal partnerships involve a joint endeavor and clearly specify the rights and responsibilities of each partner as they work toward a common goal. When public-private partnerships work, they benefit the community, the public sector, and the private sector alike.

This is the story of PROSALUD, an innovative public-private collaboration that was initiated before the term "health sector reform" was commonly used in Bolivia. Hence, it is one of the truly seminal events of the health sector reform that occurred after the economic and health care crisis in Bolivia. The crisis led to conditions that allowed this innovative approach to be dreamed of and come to fruition. This reform took place in an area where the public-sector health system was nearly nonexistent in providing necessary services.

PROSALUD and MSH have used the lessons of time, which have proven the long-term viability of this approach, to document this experience. PROSALUD is not a pilot project with only one or two years of positive results but a mature organization in its second decade of existence, which is making a difference in Bolivia. It has brought essential, high-quality health services to the underserved and others. It is a living example from which we can all learn as we face the challenges of health development in the 21st century.

The authors would like to acknowledge the following people for their contributions to PROSALUD and to this book: Antonio R. Arrázola, Zulema Gutiérrez, Martha Mérida, Luis Santa Cruz, and Pilar Sebastián (cofounders); and Roy Brooks, Aníbal Mejía, and Pamela J. Putney (long-term advisers). We would also like to thank the following people from the USAID mission in Bolivia for their contributions: Sigrid Anderson, Gerry Bowers, Paul Ehmer, Paul Hartenberger, and Lee Hougen (Health, Population, and Nutrition Officers) and Rafael Indaburu and Elba Mercado (PROSALUD's Project Officers). Thanks are also due to Jack Galloway of USAID/Ecuador and Roberto Iunes of the Inter-American Development Bank, who generously gave their time to review the book. At MSH, David Collins, Janice Miller, and Stephen Sacca read and commented on it.

The authors would also like to acknowledge Barbara Timmons for her excellent judgment in finalizing this book. In addition to editing it and managing its production, she compiled the chronology and references, and translated chapter 8.

Chronology

1982 Democracy restored in Bolivia

1983 USAID approves the Self-Financing Primary Health Care Project

1985 USAID signs agreement with Management Sciences for Health to provide technical assistance

1985 New democratically elected government takes office, launches New Economic Policy

1985 PROSALUD established

1985 Local MOH office authorizes PROSALUD to organize and operate primary health care services

1986 Bolivian government creates Fondo Social de Emergencia

1986 Municipality of Santa Cruz approves the financing of three clinics to be administered by PROSALUD

1987 PROSALUD has successfully established a network of five clinics

1987 Fondo Social de Emergencia contributes $250,000 to construct six new clinics in Santa Cruz City

1987 PROSALUD refines its delivery and financial models

1987 Opening of three new centers over 12 months

1988 First strategic planning process; referral system trial

1989 Board of Directors established

1990 First project concludes, with PROSALUD employing 90 service delivery staff members to provide primary health care in the periurban areas of Santa Cruz through a network of 15 health facilities

1991   Second five-year project funded by USAID to replicate the Santa Cruz experience in La Paz and El Alto and add a referral hospital

1993   PROSALUD opens a 25-bed hospital in Santa Cruz City as the referral center of its primary care network

1994   Enactment of legislation giving municipalities and local governments a role in the management of health facilities

1995   Beginning of national reproductive health social marketing project with Population Services International

1995   USAID financing received for further expansion of PRO-SALUD

1995   External evaluation of PROSALUD

1996   The PROSALUD network adds 14 health centers: 7 in La Paz and 7 in El Alto

1997   USAID commits endowment of $5 million

1997   By the end of the year, PROSALUD had opened 5 new health centers. The PROSALUD clinic network consisted of 32 primary health care facilities in seven cities of Bolivia and one hospital. In 1997 PROSALUD as a whole attained over 70% self-financing from user fees, with staff consultancies, grants for research activities, and training fees generating the remainder of its support.

1999   Opening of two new health centers, in Cochabamba and Oruro

1
The Private Sector and Health Reform: An Introduction

The Changing Roles of the Public and Private Sectors

Recent years have seen changes in long-standing ideological beliefs and entrenched political systems, including a dramatic shift in the attitudes of some countries toward the role of government in the economy and the society at large. Government is no longer viewed as the sole planner and supplier of all elements of economic and social life; rather the importance of individual preferences and desires has been increasingly emphasized. This shift in views holds for the health sector as well, despite the fact that this is an area where the role of government and the public sector is highly salient even in countries where the private sector's role in the economy is well established and accepted.

Government resources have not been sufficient to maintain existing health systems, meet increased demand due to population growth, increase access to services for those not covered by the current systems, and improve the quality and level of care provided. Concerns about the ability of governments to finance health services adequately, the poor performance of public health service delivery systems, and the desire to expand the choices available to patients have led a number of countries to encourage the expansion of the private sector.

Many of these countries have looked to the private sector to fill the resource gap by taking on greater responsibilities. Other countries have sought to privatize the public health system as a way of disengaging the government from the health sector, because of rising costs, public

1

dissatisfaction, and a myriad of other problems. As a result, where allowed by government policy (or lack of policy), the private sector has become a major player in the health sector. In many countries, government is no longer the main provider and financier of health services. Thus a role for the private sector in health has begun to evolve, either by design or default.

In many countries, individuals from all economic strata are increasingly using private health facilities and providers, including private hospitals, physicians, pharmacists, and traditional healers. Consumers' perception of the relative advantages of the private sector, with respect to quality of care, availability of services and drugs, amenities, location, and waiting time, has fueled much of this change in utilization patterns.

Health sector reform is occurring in both developed and developing countries as they try to determine how the health system should be organized and financed and who should benefit from it. The environment within which countries are seeking health reform often includes decreasing resources to support the public-sector elements of the health system, which has resulted in continued deterioration of public health facilities and the services they offer. This deterioration leads to further reduction in demand for services at public facilities and a transfer of that demand to the private sector.

The Necessity of Public-Private Partnerships

This book acknowledges the necessity of thinking in terms of a partnership between the public and private sectors to advance the cause of health. It is in this context that many countries are seeking strategies and solutions that will allow them to use both public and private providers and sources of financing to address the issue of improving the health of their citizens.

The objective is to use the private sector more effectively to meet public health goals by identifying policies that can improve the quality, distribution, and cost-effectiveness of the private production of health services. Although the basic economic arguments are straightforward, many aspects of the market for health services present challenges for public response that depend more on noneconomic assessments of social and political priorities. Some health services, such as public health and infectious and communicable disease management, are inherently public, since private producers will always produce too few of these services. However, for other important services, particularly acute and curative personal care, the arguments for public provision are less obvious, because the private sector can and does produce a significant proportion of these services in many settings.

In the simplest terms, the desired public-private mix is often assessed as a matter of balancing efficiency and equity considerations. From this perspective, the private sector is typically seen as being more efficient, and the public sector, as more equitable.

Countries at all economic levels are reforming their health systems to improve services and adjust to new circumstances. Recent experiences have demonstrated that public-sector policies aimed at extending access to services cannot succeed without action in the private sector. Government strategies that focus on reducing demand, improving efficiency, and generating increased revenue in the public sector generally reinforce an expanded role for private provision of services. Although it is essential to recognize the limitations of markets in meeting the public goals of equity, access, and efficiency, the public sector may fail to meet these goals. Public policy attention to these issues is equally important regardless of the relative size or market penetration of the sectors in health care delivery. However, the form in which these issues are addressed will vary and the sectors' relative roles shift. Increased recognition of private-sector roles opens the way for more effective public policy.

PROSALUD's Response to the Economic Crisis in Bolivia

In 1985, Bolivia suffered a severe economic crisis, which resulted in significant deterioration of all social-sector services, leaving a large segment of the population without access to and dissatisfied with the basic health services. It is in this context that PROSALUD came into being. A team of Bolivian professionals created an innovative health model that respects the values and cultures of the communities being served and has strong potential to become sustainable over the long term without substantial dependence on funding from external donors and to be replicated in other countries. Designed to be compatible with the goals and policies of the national health system, PROSALUD has evolved into a network of high-quality and low-cost health services, with the active participation of the communities it serves. In order to build a true public-private coalition, PROSALUD works under special agreements with the Ministry of Health and municipalities.

PROSALUD illustrates the ability of a creative, client-focused model to address key health reform issues such as quality and access and to provide a realistic, sustainable, and replicable solution to many of the problems of a health system. The history and resilience of this model give it validity. The PROSALUD model has provided a vehicle for change in Bolivia that many countries seek to emulate: it has promoted collaboration between the public and private sectors; supported innovation; identified an appropriate expansion path for private-sector services; improved information for policy and planning; and enhanced the management capacity of the health system.

This book seeks to provide information on this innovative model and encourage discussion of how such models can facilitate health reform through the use of the private sector. While each country is unique—with its own history, priorities, resources, and political context—the issues and options to address them have many similarities. But what is an effective strategy in one country may not be feasible or appropriate for another. The challenge is to not prescribe what works, but for each country to understand the conditions that made such a model effective in Bolivia. Health decision-makers in other countries can use this book to identify, for their own context, health reforms that the private and public sectors working together can achieve.

The Structure of This Book

The rest of this book is organized into eight chapters: Chapter 2 analyzes the context in which the PROSALUD public-private model was developed. Chapter 3 describes PROSALUD in detail, focusing on its mission and objectives. The strategy and structure of the organization are detailed in chapter 4, while chapter 5 focuses on its financing and long-term financial sustainability. Chapter 6 describes the achievements of PROSALUD—for example, how it has become sustainable and not just another "demonstration project" and how it has contributed to health sector reform in Bolivia.

Chapter 7 examines how the PROSALUD model was replicated in other cities in Bolivia, with an emphasis on the guiding principles that made this possible. The last two chapters of this book (chapters 8 and 9) explore the challenges that PROSALUD overcame and the key elements of its implementation, as well as the conditions that are necessary to apply the model in other countries. The conclusion discusses PRO-SALUD's future in Bolivia and its expansion to other countries, which has already begun.

2
The Context of PROSALUD's Development

The Country

Bolivia, located in the heart of South America, is culturally diverse and multilingual, sharing the problems that most countries face on the difficult road to development. In 1992, Bolivia had an estimated population of 6.5 million, concentrated in the high plain and valley regions (8.1 million as of 1999, according to IPPF). More than half of Bolivia's people reside in urban or outlying urban areas. This numerical advantage over the rural population is a manifestation of urbanization, which has accelerated in recent years. According to the country's "population pyramid," 32% of the population is economically active, 68% of the population is below the age of 20, and 41% is under 15 years of age. In 1988, the overall fertility rate was calculated at 5.0, which had declined to 4.2 by 1999 (IPPF 1999).

With its long history of political instability and recent bouts of hyperinflation, Bolivia remains one of the poorest countries in Latin America. However, the country has experienced generally improving economic conditions since market-oriented policies were introduced, which reduced inflation from 11,700% in 1985 to 9% in 1993, while the gross national product grew by an annual average of 3.25%. Economic reforms included privatization of many state enterprises.

Politically, the Decentralization and Popular Participation laws were enacted. These laws applied to the government as a whole but affected the health sector by giving more authority and resources, with community participation, to municipalities and local governments.

Health Status and Services in Bolivia

According to the National Health Policy Guidelines established by the Ministry of Health, "Bolivia is still among the countries [in Latin America] with the highest mortality levels (infant and overall). Despite a lack of reliable statistics, infant mortality rates are estimated at 102 deaths per thousand live births; by region, infant mortality is calculated at 83 per thousand in urban areas and 120 per thousand in rural areas" (Ministry of Health 1989). By 1994, according to the National Survey of Population and Health, infant mortality remained high but had declined overall to 75 per 1,000 (60 per 1,000 in urban areas and 92 per 1,000 in rural areas) (PAHO 1998).

Other data affirm the deficient status of health among the Bolivian population. For example, average life expectancy was 58 years for men and 63 for women in 1998. Child morbidity in Bolivia is twice the average for South America. Maternal mortality is also high: 390 per 100,000 live births (IPPF 1999), almost twice the regional average (United Nations 1997). Factors associated with this figure are the high fertility rate, deficiencies in maternal health care, lack of prenatal and maternity care, and a high incidence of induced abortions.

Due to the rapid growth in poor neighborhoods on the outskirts of large cities and in rural areas, malnutrition has been widespread (16% of children under five as of the 1994 DHS). Short birth intervals, along with malnutrition, contribute to the high maternal and infant mortality rates. Tuberculosis and silicosis represent other important health problems.

However, the main health care problem in Bolivia continues to be limited maternal and infant health care services. Factors related to this low level of coverage include

- the structure of public services
- lack of coordination among public and private entities
- underutilization of personnel within MOH units
- the lack of an efficient system for buying and distributing medicine and medical supplies
- deficiencies in ongoing training of medical, paramedical, and administrative personnel

- lack of financial resources
- cultural barriers.

The Public and Private Health Sectors in Bolivia

It is estimated that only one-third of the Bolivian population is receiving adequate medical attention (USAID 1999). In 1988, only 20% of the pregnant women in the areas of El Alto, La Paz, Cochabamba, and Santa Cruz received prenatal care, while postnatal coverage reached just 6%. Fewer than one in every five families in the area under coverage received a visit during the same period by personnel from the MOH or any other institution. Secondary and tertiary services were available to an even smaller proportion of the population. Much of the lack of coverage was due to poor communication and lack of coordination among the extension services offered by health centers, reference services, and hospitals. Such limited overall coverage has led to the growth of nongovernmental organizations and the practice of nontraditional medicine. In the outlying areas of the country's major cities, the public health care system, especially at the primary level, was barely visible. Consequently, the responsibility has fallen upon mothers' clubs and other community organizations to undertake the important tasks of food distribution, nutrition, and other services related to child survival.

In 1993, the MOH provided services to 43% of the national population (47% in urban areas and 39% in rural areas), while the private sector (including traditional providers and private pharmacies) provided 46% of health services (43% in urban areas and 48% in rural areas). Figure 1 shows the sources of care according to location of population.

The public sector is composed of the traditional MOH services and the government-run Health Insurance Plan (Cajas de Salud or Social Security) clinics. Administratively, the MOH comprises a central level, regional offices, and health districts. Health centers, district hospitals, and reference hospitals (tertiary level) make up the health care delivery system. Since 1995, municipalities and local governments have played a role in the management of health facilities.

The private sector includes for-profit and nonprofit components. The for-profit health services are characterized by

Figure 1. Urban and Rural Health Coverage by Provider Type

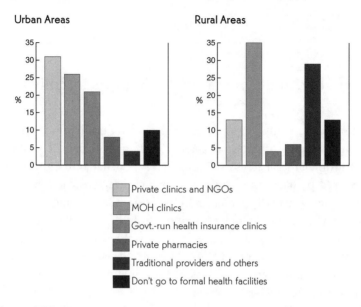

Source: MOH 1993.

- a primarily curative orientation
- personnel with multiple professional commitments (both private and public)
- limited access determined by the cost of services and clients' ability to pay
- financial and administrative management problems
- limited equipment
- low coverage
- urban locations
- dependence on its own financial resources
- lack of integration into the national health care system.

The private nonprofit sector is heterogeneous and not well organized. It is characterized by

- a charitable orientation
- low-cost or free services

- location in outlying urban areas
- difficulties in administration
- preventive and treatment-oriented services, with outreach at various levels
- dependence on outside funding
- work not tied to the national health care system.

Changes in the Environment

The watershed year for Bolivia was 1985, when it began to reform its political and economic systems. The following sections give an overview of the social, political, and economic changes and their effects on the health sector and the start-up of PROSALUD.

The Context before 1985
Democracy restored after years of military dictatorship. Bolivia had suffered from political instability for decades. In 1982, after a very difficult process, a democratic government was installed as part of a national consensus to return to democracy. The governing coalition, the Unidad Democrática y Popular, had the difficult task of managing a damaged economy while maintaining satisfied trade unions and other social groups wishing to enjoy the immediate results of this newly born democracy.

Severe political and economic crisis. Political problems, exacerbated by the economic crisis that began at the end of the 1970s, pushed the country into hyperinflation and recession between 1982 and 1985. The economic policy was characterized by a "terrible divorce with reality" and caused the most severe economic crisis in Bolivian history. Per capita income dropped by more than one-third and hyperinflation worsened the already weak economy. The inflation rate in the first quarter of 1985 reached 26,000%, the highest in the Western Hemisphere and the seventh in the world (Nogales 1989).

Significant deterioration of the social sector. The economic recession seriously eroded the Bolivian government's ability to adequately finance social-sector activities. From 1980 to 1987, the percentage of the budget allotted to health care fell dramatically, from 8% of the gross national product in 1981 to 2% in 1986. To cope with this, the health sector fundamentally restructured the financing of the MOH, which had accounted for about 90% of total national spending on health. As a result of the crisis, MOH financing slipped to between 50 and 60%, with devastating effects on the quality and accessibility of health services for low-income populations. The budget was complemented by a combination of external assistance and user fees for some services. Most of the MOH funds, approximately 88%, were spent on personnel, leaving an insufficient amount for supplies, equipment, and drugs. In addition, salaries fell significantly in real terms throughout this period. This resulted in low motivation and strong reactions from trade unions. Absenteeism and tardiness were high and exacerbated by long periods of strikes (Fiedler 1990).

The events discussed above had four major effects on the health sector and its organization and financing:

- *Increased community participation:* During 1982–85, the MOH launched an ambitious health program, which incorporated primary health care and community participation for the first time ever. This process, led by Minister of Health Javier Torres Goytia, raised awareness and provided a unique opportunity for the population to become part of the solution of its own health problems. In this period, massive community mobilizations contributed significantly to increase immunization against preventable diseases. The concept of primary health care started to be implemented in the country for the first time. Historically these should be recognized as the first attempts to reform the sector.

- *Deteriorating quality of public services:* Despite these efforts, the severe economic crisis affected the government's health program. Because of both the economic recession and the change in the use of the meager resources, the quality of services suffered significantly, leaving many people without access to and dissatisfied with basic health care services.

- *Public-sector fees for services:* It was impossible for the MOH to provide free services at previous levels. To cope with this situation, most public services relied on revenues from unofficial user fees to keep services running. Although it was not an established policy, charging fees became a necessity for public hospitals and health centers, to compensate for the drastic reduction in government funding.

- *Public demand for affordable alternatives:* To meet their health needs, low- to middle-income people started to demand affordable alternatives. By 1985, at the end of this acute recession, the quality of public services was very low and private services were unaffordable for most people.

The Watershed: After 1985

The year 1985 is remembered in Bolivia because major changes took place to overcome the worst political and economic crisis in its history. The most important were the election of a democratic government, the New Economic Policy, and structural adjustments. These events and some resulting social problems are briefly described below.

- *Consolidation of democratic government:* Forced out by the economic recession, the government left office one year before its term ended. On August 6, 1985, a new, democratically elected government took office, with the promise to fight hyperinflation and implement fundamental changes in the economy of the country.

- *New economic order:* The newly elected democratic government launched its New Economic Policy (NEP) on August 29, 1985. The implementation of this policy enabled the government to put an end to the hyperinflationary period and reorient the roles and functions of the public and private sectors. The NEP was a dramatic and sudden change in macroeconomic policies and was attained by drastic changes in regulations and in the way the economy was handled. In sum, the NEP changed "the rules of the game" by establishing a free market economy. The impact of these measures on the gross domestic product is shown in Figure 2.

- *Structural adjustments:* As a part of the NEP, Bolivia started a structural adjustment program in 1985, which changed the role and functions of the state and opened up new opportunities for the private sector. The government took drastic measures to reduce the fiscal deficit, including reducing the size of the public sector through privatization from 1989 to 1997, decreasing the number of public employees, and improving taxation systems.

- *Emerging social problems:* The NEP and other coincidental conditions produced social problems that challenged the new structures. Unemployment caused by the closing of state-owned mines

Figure 2. The Impact of the New Economic Policy on the Gross Domestic Product

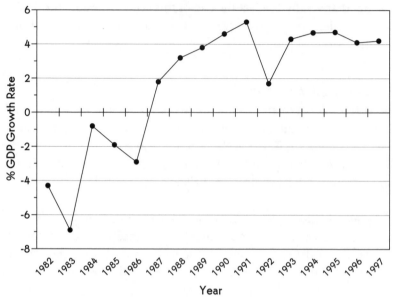

and problems in agriculture, and the economic recession forced migration to cities, increased the importance of the so-called informal sector of the economy, and contributed to the increase in demand for health and other social services, such as education and housing. (The informal sector is composed of unsalaried, casual laborers, or self-employed workers such as taxi drivers and street vendors.)

Effects on the Health Sector: A New Paradigm

The government's neoliberal policies permitted structural changes in the economy. Despite serious social costs, economic stability was achieved. However, the recession was not completely overcome, and the social sector (health, education, and housing) was especially affected. The main result of the process begun in 1985 was a new paradigm for Bolivian society and therefore for the health sector that cleared the way for the health sector reform that started in 1990. Its new principles were emphasis on local government, modernization of the social sector, opportunities for the private sector, new criteria for external aid, and new health financing mechanisms, as detailed below.

- *Emphasis on local government:* The passage of the Decentralization and Popular Participation laws in 1994 changed the role of the central government and provided new responsibilities for municipalities and local governments in the administration and financing of health and other social services.

- *Modernization of the social sector:* Once the major changes were implemented in the economic sector, a process of modernization of the social sector started in 1989. Educational reform took the lead, and after a long process of political negotiations, began to be implemented in 1995. Taking a more conservative approach, the health sector started its modernization process in 1990. The major changes in the health sector are attributable to broad structural changes such as the Decentralization Law and the Popular Participation Law.

- *Opportunities for the private sector:* From 1989 on, the government officially recognized and highlighted the importance of the private sector, both for-profit and nonprofit, and incorporated it into the National Health Policy. The increased participation of the private sector in the provision of health care was needed to reduce the burden of the still weak public sector and was congruent with the government's overall policy. In practice, the MOH signed agreements with various nongovernmental organizations to formalize and coordinate health care programs in both rural and urban areas. In 1994, the Popular Participation Law brought new opportunities to the nongovernmental sector to provide public health services through contracts with municipalities and decentralized MOH districts.

- *New criteria for external aid:* In November 1986, the government created the Fondo Social de Emergencia (FSE), a "safety net" to channel soft loans to support social programs. The FSE was established as an autonomous institution, staffed with technical personnel and free of political pressures. It established a new mindset for both social investment and external aid in Bolivia. In 1987, its first year of operations, the FSE approved 460 social projects for private agencies (nongovernmental organizations, neighborhood organizations, churches, cooperatives) and public agencies (local governments, municipalities) and invested $37.2 million. In 1998, the FSE approved 1,657 projects representing an investment of $116.9 million. In 1987, PROSALUD was one of the institutions that received $250,000 to support the construction of six clinics in Santa Cruz City on land provided by the mayor's office.

Scarce resources from public and foreign assistance were focused on priority problems. As funding became more difficult to obtain, the FSE and most other donors introduced new criteria to both governmental and nongovernmental recipients. Cost-effectiveness, efficiency, community participation, transparency, focus on results, and concerns about sustainability became standard terms and conditions.

- *New health financing mechanisms:* The government started charging user fees in 1983, partially shifting the responsibility for financing care from the MOH to the public. From 1984 to 1988, revenues from user fees grew by more than 600%, from $1.7 million to $10.3 million. In La Paz, Cochabamba, and Santa Cruz, the three main *departamentos* (provinces) of Bolivia, the proportion of total public hospital budget resources from user fees grew from 13% in 1984 to 40% in 1988. MOH expenditure in 1987 stood at less than half (46%) of its 1980 level (38% of its 1980 level in per capita terms). In 1996 the MOH and municipalities jointly launched the National Insurance for Mothers and Children program (Seguro Nacional de Maternidad y Niñez, or SNMN) to increase access to health services for low-income populations. These initiatives are expected to continue as a part of the health sector reform process.

Factors That Contributed to the Development of PROSALUD

Many elements of the changing political and economic situation in Bolivia and the reform of its health sector contributed to creating an environment within which PROSALUD, begun in 1985, could develop and grow:

- *Donor support and technical assistance:* Crucial to the development and implementation of PROSALUD were the financial support and guidance of the US Agency for International Development (USAID/Bolivia mission representatives in the Office of Health and Human Resources) and technical assistance from Management Sciences for Health.

- *New economic policies:* The downturn in the economy had a substantial impact on the health sector, as evidenced by a reduction in the quality of public services. Persistent economic and infrastructure problems can also be blamed for the absence of a primary health care service network in rural and outlying urban areas. New economic policies contributed to the development of PROSALUD by fostering monetary stability and favorable conditions for private initiatives.

- *Willingness to pay for quality services:* Another factor was the public's willingness to contribute financially to maintaining the system in exchange for high-quality, low-cost services.

- *Legislation favoring participatory government:* Decentralization and the renewed democratization of municipal governments fostered broader participation in health concerns.

- *Experimentation:* One of the factors contributing to the development of PROSALUD was the willingness of the Bolivian government, through the MOH, to experiment with a new plan for providing health care in order to broaden coverage.

- *Growth of the informal sector:* People who work in the informal sector generally have lower incomes than those in the formal sector and benefit from the kinds of services PROSALUD offers (for example, free preventive care). Consequently, the increase in the number of people working in the informal sector contributed to PROSALUD's growth.

- *Political support:* During the USAID-funded project (which began in 1983—see chapter 3), the firm and lasting support of regional authorities, both civilian and political, was important. The strong backing of the beneficiary communities, after promotion of grassroots involvement ("animation"), was equally significant. The FSE and the regional health office and city government of Santa Cruz also played important roles by providing or financing the health care infrastructure and by placing their confidence in PROSALUD.

- *Health policy paradigm shift:* Finally, conceptual changes in national health policy, such as adherence to the principles of good management, decentralization, and focus on maternal and child health care, and acknowledgment of the need to work with the private sector, were also significant.

3

What Is PROSALUD?

It is not enough to create a functioning health system which cannot
survive over the long term without substantial donor assistance. The
real challenge is to establish the mechanisms that will ensure a sustainable health system for communities with scarce resources.
                                        —PROSALUD's strategic plan, 1988

In response to growing needs in the health sector, in 1985 a team of
Bolivian professionals created PROSALUD (the Asociación Protección
a la Salud), with financing from the US Agency for International Development and technical assistance from Management Sciences for Health.
This health care model provides self-financing, sustainable health care
that is compatible with national health policies and the population's
needs.

PROSALUD is a network of health services serving low-income and
lower-middle class populations in urban and periurban areas. Legally
it is a private, nonprofit Bolivian health care organization. As of the
end of 1999, it offers services to about half a million people in nine
cities throughout the country, with headquarters in Santa Cruz. This
chapter describes its philosophy and functions, the population it serves,
and its history.

The Mission and Values of PROSALUD

In 1988, PROSALUD conducted a strategic planning process, which produced the organization's first long-term vision and a conceptual framework that defined the main barriers to providing self-financing health
services, the strategies to address these obstacles, and the project's long-

VISION

"PROSALUD will be a sustainable national organization, leader, and alternative in the delivery of high-quality and low-cost health care services and products."

MISSION

The mission of PROSALUD is "to support human development by contributing to the health and well-being of the population, especially those with few resources."

MOTTO

"*Su salud ante todo*" (their health above all) synthesizes the philosophy of PROSALUD and reminds all employees to be accountable to those who trust them with their health.

CORE VALUES

PROSALUD works to serve the community—without discrimination—and its work is based on the following core values:

- *Participación (participation):* Employees and beneficiaries are responsible for and play an active part in planning and decision-making.
- *Respeto (respect):* All activities shall respect the culture and reflect the values of the community in which we work.
- *Organización (organization):* All activities shall be conducted to work toward greater efficiency, effectiveness, and excellence.
- *Solidaridad (solidarity):* Our behavior should reflect our sense of service, favoring those most in need.
- *Autonomía (autonomy):* The institution is guided only by its work philosophy and governance mechanisms.
- *Legalidad (legality):* All decisions shall be made and actions taken within the law and in accordance with moral principles and shall be transparent.
- *Unidad (unity):* We are committed to work as a team to practice our principles and achieve our objectives.
- *Disciplina (discipline):* We are committed to quality work and assume personal responsibility for our actions.

RIGHTS OF USERS OF PROSALUD SERVICES

All users of services are clients and have the following rights:

- dignity
- information
- confidentiality
- quality

Source: "El libro azul de PROSALUD" ("The Blue Book of PROSALUD," an employees' handbook), pp. 3, 5, 6, 17.

term objectives. Since this was the first experience with strategic planning, the core team closely followed a planning methodology used by MSH to reach consensus on the basics: vision, mission, motto, core values, guiding principles, and general strategy. As the usefulness of these basic components and principles became more evident, they were redefined to make them more functional and easier to communicate at all levels of the organization.

Target Population

The target population of PROSALUD is composed of lower- to middle-income Bolivians in periurban areas who are relatively underserved or not served by the public and private health sectors. Typically, users of PROSALUD services are the working poor and part of the informal sector of the economy. They tend to be self-employed and therefore not covered by the Cajas de Salud, the government-run health plan for formal employees, who represent only 20% of the population.

What PROSALUD Does

The PROSALUD model strives to merge social concerns and public health objectives with private-sector initiatives. This model provides largely self-financing, sustainable health care to its target population and is compatible with both national health policy objectives and the population's needs. In addition to providing health care, PROSALUD performs several important functions, identified as its strategic activities:

- *Health services:* PROSALUD's core business is providing high-quality primary health care services.
- *Social marketing:* PROSALUD operates a national social marketing program, which sells condoms and birth control pills to clients at low cost through the commercial sector, including nontraditional outlets.
- *Training:* PROSALUD offers training in health services administration and in the design, implementation, and management of health programs, focusing on maternal/child health, family planning, and quality assurance.

- *Research:* In order to better understand and approach the major health problems in communities, PROSALUD regularly carries out marketing, epidemiological, and operations research, often in collaboration with national and international organizations.

- *Technical assistance:* PROSALUD provides technical assistance to other health organizations in Bolivia and other countries. PRO-SALUD's staff members have provided technical assistance in Brazil, Ecuador, Guatemala, Haiti, Honduras, Kenya, Nicaragua, Paraguay, Uruguay, and Zambia.

Who PROSALUD Serves

PROSALUD is a client-oriented, primary health care-centered delivery system distinguished by its ability to provide a high volume of high-quality and affordable services with high levels of efficiency, self-financing, and patient satisfaction. Over 580 PROSALUD employees working in 33 clinics and a 25-bed referral hospital provide health care services to approximately 500,000 lower- to middle-income people a year.

How PROSALUD Is Financed

PROSALUD provides all preventive services, roughly half of all of its care, free of charge. It charges relatively low prices, only slightly higher than those levied by MOH facilities, for curative services. Additionally, roughly 10% of all the curative services delivered by PROSALUD are provided free to indigent clients. PROSALUD's health network recuperates over 70% of its costs from user fees. This represents one of the highest levels of self-sufficiency in the developing world, a noteworthy achievement in a country considered the second poorest in Latin America.

Chapter 5 describes PROSALUD's financial model, which uses cross-subsidies as well as user fees. The financial support of USAID (for the project described below and the endowment) made the organization's founding and expansion possible.

Although salaried employees provide most services, PROSALUD controls costs by paying specialist physicians (such as pediatricians, obstetrician/gynecologists, and dentists) on a fee-sharing basis instead of paying them salaries. In return for a share of the revenues generated by the specialist, PROSALUD provides consulting rooms, a high volume of patients, and management support at both the clinic and headquarters.

How PROSALUD Is Managed

The National Office houses the Management Support Unit, which oversees systems development, marketing, and planning and administers the PROSALUD network, including

- hiring and training personnel
- purchasing and distributing drugs and supplies
- establishing working relationships with other services providers in the area, including the MOH
- managing community relations
- maintaining the fiscal and financial structures
- overseeing the delivery of services and controlling quality.

The departments of Finance, Medical Services, Marketing, Training, and Development are also located in the central office. Two critical elements of PROSALUD's management system are its use of a data-driven monitoring, evaluation, and planning system and its personnel recruitment criteria, process, and training plan.

How PROSALUD Developed

Although PROSALUD has undergone several phases of development, its goal has remained the same: to establish a sustainable and cost-effective private-sector alternative for the delivery of primary health care services, targeted to the low-income population in urban and periurban areas of Bolivia.

Phase One, 1983–85: Creation of PROSALUD

In November 1983, the US Agency for International Development (USAID) approved the Self-Financing Primary Health Care Project. The project was initially designed to serve an identified population of cooperatives (rural and urban). Its objective was to demonstrate that health care could be provided on a self-financing basis through a prepayment model. However, in early 1985, the cooperatives concluded that they could not reach a workable agreement and withdrew from the project.

The relationship with the cooperatives failed in part because the project was designed in isolation from the community. This lack of participation resulted in each group having its own agenda, which did not correspond to the project's stated objectives. In addition, the assumption that the cooperatives provided a captive audience that would use the health care centers was never adequately investigated.

The withdrawal of the cooperatives triggered a process of redefining the managerial and operational structure of the project and reconceptualizing its objectives and design. The project evolved into a network of community-sponsored health centers, directed by the Management Support Unit of PROSALUD.

In 1985, USAID executed an agreement with Management Sciences for Health to assist with running the Management Support Unit and coordinating technical assistance. MSH and USAID agreed that a private, independent organization should replace the cooperatives as the principal implementer of the project. On August 21, 1985, PROSALUD was legally formed as a nonprofit organization to replace the cooperatives as the Management Support Unit for the primary health care delivery system.

Phase Two, 1985–91: Implementation of the PROSALUD Model

Identifying "customers" willing to participate in the project as cosponsors of the primary health care services and marketing partners for the self-financing initiatives became a central consideration for the project. PROSALUD conducted intense promotional activities in the periurban and rural communities surrounding Santa Cruz and established relationships with municipal governments and community organizations.

In October 1985, the Santa Cruz office of the MOH authorized PROSALUD to organize and operate primary health care services. After much negotiation with several community organizations, PROSALUD opened two health centers in Santa Cruz. PROSALUD hired personnel and installed the necessary equipment while each community provided the building. Subsequently, PROSALUD signed an agreement with the municipality that led to the opening of three new centers in 1987–88. In 1988, the Fondo Social de Emergencia made a significant contribution to construct six new centers.

In April 1989, PROSALUD established a Board of Directors. It is composed of prominent citizens who meet regularly to review PRO-SALUD's activities, provide guidance, discuss new opportunities, and approve the budget.

At the conclusion of the first project in August 1990, PROSALUD was providing primary health care in the periurban areas of Santa Cruz through a network of 15 health facilities, with 90 service delivery staff members and a Management Support Unit of 19 people involved in operations management, quality assurance, and logistics.

Phase Three, 1991–97: Growth of PROSALUD

In May 1991, the organization embarked on a new five-year plan funded by USAID to replicate the Santa Cruz experience in the La Paz metropolitan area and add a referral center (hospital) in Santa Cruz. By the end of 1996, the PROSALUD network had added 14 health centers: 7 in La Paz and 7 in El Alto (in the La Paz metropolitan area). After the centers in El Alto were set up, it was recognized that the community was significantly poorer than Santa Cruz, and thus additional centers were opened in La Paz to cross-subsidize the less sustainable centers in El Alto. In Santa Cruz, the secondary care 25-bed hospital has operated since August 1993 to support the primary health care network. PRO-SALUD was the direct and sole grantee of the $6.5 million cooperative agreement with USAID that supported the opening of this hospital, and it subcontracted technical assistance as needed.

Another expansion of PROSALUD occurred in 1995 with USAID financing, to support the health sector reform movement in Bolivia. Under this project, additional health centers were planned for various parts of the country. By the end of 1997, PROSALUD had opened two new health centers in the communities of Tarija (south), one in Yacuiba (south), one in Riberalta (north), and one in Puerto Quijarro (east). In addition, PROSALUD opened new health centers in Cochabamba and Oruro cities at the end of 1999.

To adapt to this growth, PROSALUD's organizational structure grew to include decentralized Regional Offices to manage health centers. The National Office began to set the organization's policies, respond to requests for PROSALUD services, and provide technical assistance both domestically and internationally. Staff members from the National Office traveled to different countries to share PROSALUD's cost recovery health care model.

As the delivery model was replicated in very different settings, it was modified to respond to different environments and address the lessons learned along the way (see chapter 8 and the conclusion). As a result of this "cross-fertilization," the concept of a basic health center evolved into polyclinics, and more ambulatory services were added to existing and new facilities. PROSALUD also adapted its management information system to integrate accounting, management, and patient statistics software systems.

Phase Four, 1997–99 and the Future: PROSALUD's Impact

By the end of 2002, USAID will have invested approximately $14 million in PROSALUD, of which about 10% was for technical assistance. By the end of the century, PROSALUD will be on the verge of financial self-sustainability and will be providing high-quality, low-cost services to more than half a million low- and lower-middle-income Bolivians (Holley 1996).

PROSALUD has evolved over the past 14 years to become a significant force in the health care sector in Bolivia. It has demonstrated that high-quality health care can be provided to low-income populations at affordable prices and that financial self-sustainability is possible. In the process, it has developed service delivery models and managerial expertise that will guarantee its success in the future, and it has repeatedly demonstrated the high degree of commitment required of its staff to develop and carry out complex projects with international funding.

PROSALUD has had a significant impact on both the public and private health care sectors in Bolivia. The Bolivian MOH has adopted several elements of the PROSALUD model, including 24-hour medical service, risk-sharing with specialists (fee-sharing arrangements), and proactive social marketing campaigns. In the private commercial sector, the change is even more noticeable. To better compete with PRO-SALUD's high-quality care and low costs, prices have fallen and the quality of services has improved. The midterm evaluation of PRO-SALUD conducted by POPTECH for USAID (Fiedler and Hougen

1995) identified these indirect effects on the health care market as perhaps the most important and enduring benefits of the project. Furthermore, the evaluation highlighted the need to measure and quantify
these effects.

The ability to replicate the PROSALUD model in areas that differ
culturally, geographically, and economically has already been demonstrated in Bolivia. The model has been reproduced successfully in eight
cities throughout the country and continues to expand rapidly, with
each new center being carefully modified according to the unique environment in which it operates. Chapter 7 provides details on how and
where the PROSALUD experience has been replicated.

4

PROSALUD's Structure, Systems, and Services

Organizational Governance and Structure

PROSALUD is governed by an Assembly of Associates, Board of Directors, National Office (headquarters), Regional Offices, and the Health Services Network. PROSALUD's "Manual of Organization and Functions" describes the basic organization shown in Figure 3.

Assembly of Associates

The highest authority is the Assembly of Associates. It is responsible for determining the overall policies of the organization and generally overseeing the work of the board and executives of PROSALUD. The Assembly of Associates is composed of the board members (six), former board members, founding nonsalaried members, members of the National Executive Committee, and six associates who will be future board members.

Board of Directors

The board is elected by the nonsalaried members of the Assembly and acts as its representative. It formulates and approves policies, receives and reviews reports from the Executive Director, approves pricing policies, and in general oversees the functioning of the organization. The Endowment Committee is a special body created to manage and control the capital assets, certificates, and other securities that constitute the endowment fund, and the income, interest dividends, and/or capital gains that are produced.

Figure 3. Organization of PROSALUD

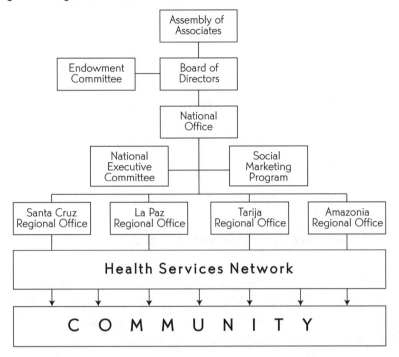

National Office
The National Office provides overall executive direction to PROSALUD but has little to do with day-to-day operations. It is responsible for

- organizational planning and development
- coordination and support of the Regional Offices
- monitoring and evaluation of services
- coordination of broad functions such as finance, marketing, and quality assurance
- project development
- liaison with the international and local communities.

Regional Offices
The Regional Offices oversee the Health Services Network. They function autonomously and are responsible for the following broad areas:

- managing and supporting the clinic network

- managing the health care delivery system
- ensuring community participation

Each Regional Office has a Director and a team of professionals organized into various departments. These departments structure their systems to support the production of services. The support systems consist of supplies, maintenance, transportation, supervision, training, marketing, personnel administration, and management information systems. PROSALUD's organizational manual clearly spells out the decision-making authority of the Regional Offices. These offices coordinate activities with district health authorities and provide service and epidemiological data for the districts' health information systems.

National Executive Committee
The National Executive Committee is a coordinating and technical body composed of the staff of the National Office and the Directors of the Regional Offices. It meets three or four times a year to evaluate progress against work plans and to formulate the strategic plan.

Health Services Network
The Health Services Network is composed of clinics and, in the case of Santa Cruz, includes a hospital. Each has a Medical Director and a professional team supervised by the respective Regional Office. A primary objective of PROSALUD is to build managerial capabilities at the clinic level.

PROSALUD clinics provide an integrated, comprehensive, and continuous package of basic preventive and curative health care. Clinics also serve as outlets for socially marketed products.

There are two types of clinics: basic clinics and polyclinics. Polyclinics offer a broader range of services than basic clinics and act as referral facilities for certain diagnostic and laboratory procedures. The Regional Offices operate radio communications with all the clinics in the network and serve as bases for the 24-hour ambulance service provided to network clinics.

Clinics are responsible for

- delivering high-quality health services to the community
- providing health education and other outreach activities
- ensuring a direct interface with the local community

The last item is important because one of the pillars of PROSALUD's success has been its integration into the life of communities and its responsiveness to communities' needs.

By the end of 1999, the PROSALUD clinic network consisted of 33 primary health care facilities distributed in nine cities of Bolivia and one 25-bed hospital in Santa Cruz City (see Figure 4). Each clinic served a catchment population of approximately 15,000, for a total beneficiary population of 500,000.

The PROSALUD Health Care Delivery Model

PROSALUD's health care delivery model uses clinics to provide health services in a network of decentralized, multipurpose facilities that provide integrated and comprehensive care. The box summarizes key characteristics of the clinic network.

PROSALUD clinics are

- *decentralized:* Clinics are located strategically to make them accessible to the population, and they enjoy a high degree of autonomy in their operations.

- *multipurpose:* Clinics are staffed and equipped to respond to the most common health needs and demands.

- *always open:* All clinics and the ambulance service operate 24 hours a day, 365 days a year.

The care provided in PROSALUD clinics is

- *integrated:* Preventive and curative services are interconnected to achieve greater effectiveness and efficiency. Integration means that the same staff, during the same hours and in the same facility, can provide preventive and curative services. Although integrated, priority programs do not lose their identities.

- *comprehensive:* Providers are taught to see clients as people and to take into account their environment, habits, and beliefs.

- *continuous:* There are mechanisms to ensure the follow-up of clients, especially those with needs or conditions that require con-

Figure 4. PROSALUD Health Services Network

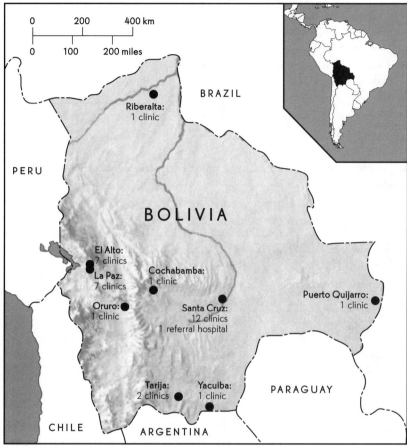

tinuity of the intervention (for example, tuberculosis, family planning, high blood pressure, and diabetes).

The outputs expected from clinics providing this form of health
care are

* *high-quality* health services
* services produced in sufficiently *high volume* to maximize efficiency and productivity
* at *low unit cost*, resulting in affordable prices for clients.

KEY CHARACTERISTICS OF THE PROSALUD CLINIC NETWORK

- The same services are provided in all basic clinics. Expanded services are offered in polyclinics. All clinics offer emergency services 24 hours a day. (See Table 1.)
- All clinics have pharmacies, delivery rooms, waiting rooms, and reception rooms; lab services and diagnostic facilities are shared among clinics.
- Clinics' physical layouts are standardized.
- Clinics have the same basic staffing pattern, but the number of staff varies by volume of patients.
- User fees are charged for curative services.
- All preventive care and priority public health services are provided free of charge.
- Clinics operate as outlets for socially marketed products.
- Clinic directors are general practioners who also provide care.

ARRANGEMENTS WITH NONSALARIED SPECIALISTS

- PROSALUD provides consultation rooms.
- Dentists provide their own equipment and supplies.
- Practitioners adhere to PROSALUD procedures and quality standards.
- Specialists split fees with PROSALUD.
- Community health workers promote clinic services, educate target population, and ensure that treatment is completed.

Services

PROSALUD clinics offer a wide range of services (see Table 1). A standardized package of essential, curative, and specialty services was defined using the government's guidelines and considering local community needs and demand. All clinics provide preventive care and other priority public health interventions free of charge. Curative and other specialty services are provided for a fee, set at levels that are affordable to the target group.

Each clinic has consultation and delivery rooms, a pharmacy, and reception/waiting areas. All clinics must comply with a physical layout that includes requirements for size and appearance (colors, decoration). Pharmacies attached to clinics sell generic drugs and other supplies. Some clinics share laboratory and diagnostic services and have

Table 1. Services Available at PROSALUD Clinics

Services Subject to Fees	*Services Exempt from Fees*
Basic clinics	
Curative consultations by general practitioners, pediatricians, and gynecologists	Immunizations
	Well-baby clinical services
	Preventive dental care
Curative dental care	Reproductive health counseling
Deliveries	Follow-up prenatal care
Initial prenatal visit	TB treatment
Family planning: all reversible methods	Malaria treatment
	Oral rehydration therapy
Nursing procedures (e.g., IV fluids)	Home visits
Emergency services (24 hours)	Health education
Pharmacy	
Polyclinics	
In addition to the above:	Immunizations
Double pediatrician and gynecologist consulting time	Well-baby clinical services
	Preventive dental care
Other specialized services: cardiology, ear/nose/throat, ophthalmology, internal medicine	Reproductive health counseling
	Postpartum care
	Follow-up prenatal care
Specialized laboratory services	TB treatment
Sonograms	Malaria treatment
Ambulatory surgery	Oral rehydration therapy
Voluntary surgical contraception (in some)	Home visits
	Health education
Hospital	
In addition to the services provided in the polyclinics:	Immunizations
	Well-baby clinical services
Surgery: Cesarean section and other simple surgical procedures	Preventive dental care
	Reproductive health counseling
Inpatient services	Postpartum care
X-ray	Follow-up prenatal care
Endoscopy	TB treatment
Specialized laboratory services, including test for HIV	Malaria treatment
	Oral rehydration therapy
Voluntary surgical contraception	Home visits
	Health education

access to ambulance services. Clinics communicate with each other via radio or telephone.

In addition to clinic-based providers, there is a minimum of one salaried community health worker (CHW) attached to each clinic. This CHW increases awareness among community members of PROSALUD clinic locations, hours, and services. Furthermore, CHWs provide basic preventive health education, including family planning, and ensure that patients, such as those receiving treatment for tuberculosis, complete their treatment.

Special Services

Eye care program. Recognizing that uncorrected refractive errors are a major cause of visual disability in low-income populations, PROSALUD implemented an eye care program. The services provided include measurement of visual errors, prescriptions for glasses, and supply of inexpensive glasses through a central optical lab. Help the World See, a nonprofit organization based in the US, has provided financial and technical support for this program.

Physical rehabilitation program. With the financial and technical assistance of De Vaal Foundation in the Netherlands, PROSALUD set up a comprehensive physical rehabilitation program in Santa Cruz and Riberalta. The services provided are physiotherapy and supply of orthopedic devices made in PROSALUD's own workshop. De Vaal Foundation covers the expenses of providing this specialized care for children with poliomyelitis and osteomyelitis, while PROSALUD markets physiotherapy services and products to other clients as an additional source of revenue.

Referral Relationships

The PROSALUD clinics are by definition the primary level of contact with the community and their basic function is to provide quality services—*including referrals to other health organizations*—within and outside PROSALUD. Foreseeing that there would be cases that could not be diagnosed or treated within the system, PROSALUD designed and tested a referral policy for patients in 1988. Some findings of the referral system test were:

- Relationships between patients and providers were often disrupted when patients were sent outside the PROSALUD system.

- Payment problems became an issue once patients were referred to more expensive facilities, particularly hospitals.

- Some patients resisted going to a public hospital because they did not trust the quality of care in public hospitals. They could afford primary care visits at PROSALUD, but they could not necessarily afford inpatient stays at private hospitals.

- If patients received satisfactory care at the more expensive tertiary care centers, the patients tended to assume that the care was more sophisticated than that at the health care clinics and would go on to seek their primary care at the tertiary facility.

- If a PROSALUD provider referred a patient to an external facility, and the patient received unsatisfactory care, the patient tended to look outside the PROSALUD system for future care.

This test resulted in an informal referral system, based principally on relations with other physicians and organizations. This trial was followed by an operations research study, which found that approximately 15% of PROSALUD users had to be referred outside the system. It became apparent that a diagnostic, evaluation, and treatment center was needed for both ambulatory and acute patients who required surgery or short-term admission.

PROSALUD conducted a feasibility study in 1991 and decided to augment its delivery capacity by opening a hospital as a referral center to respond to the unmet demands most often manifested by the community and contribute to the efficiency of the referral system—both in terms of patient satisfaction and cost to the patient in time and out-of-pocket expense. The relationships with the public hospital system still exist, since not all health problems can be resolved within the PRO-SALUD system, and formal links are still needed, even though fewer patients are referred to the public hospitals.

The PROSALUD hospital in Santa Cruz is the referral center of the primary care network. Currently the hospital is recovering in excess of 100% of its costs and using these surpluses to subsidize operations at some of the health centers and to enable PROSALUD to offer a fuller range of services, including secondary care.

Human Resources Management

Principles of Managing Staff

Recognizing that human resources were critical to the success of PRO-SALUD, the organization set as a priority the nurture of its human resources. It established the principle that if PROSALUD personnel were treated well they would treat the users of services well. PROSALUD implemented a human resources policy to avoid discrimination, corruption, and violation of human rights. To avoid these practices and, most importantly, to develop its human resources in a sustainable way, PROSALUD established the following policies:

- *Merit-based selection process:* A manual contains job descriptions and requirements for each position. In each case, the supervisor leads the process and needs participation from staff one level up and one level down to make a final decision.

- *Equal job opportunity:* Ethnic, social, gender, political, and religious discrimination is prevented through clear information to applicants, who are informed about their rights and encouraged to report and file a complaint if appropriate.

- *Job stability:* The permanence of an employee depends on performance, adherence to principles, and accountability. Employees are evaluated on a regular basis and are informed about their rights.

- *Career opportunities:* Existing employees are the first choice to fill new positions and vacancies. As a national network, PROSALUD offers employees career opportunities through internal promotion. Over the years, these have included opportunities to contribute to replicating PROSALUD in new settings.

- *Teamwork and participation:* Experiencing teamwork teaches responsibility, self-discipline, and commitment to common goals. Through teamwork all personnel have the opportunity to participate in planning, monitoring, and evaluation.

- *Training opportunities:* All personnel have not only the opportunity but also the obligation of keeping themselves up to date. All job descriptions clearly spell out the minimum number of hours that each employee should devote to training. Training is required of clinical staff to maintain and improve their technical skills. Ancillary service staff and administrative staff also receive training to improve existing job skills and develop new skills. This training in new skills allows cross-training of staff, which in turn permits managers to enhance staff productivity.

- *Compensation and incentives:* Salaries follow an explicit compensation policy based on the economic capacity of the organization and the market. A monetary and nonmonetary incentive system is part of the strategy to motivate the staff. In the early years, a portion of the revenues was distributed to employees, but this system was discontinued due to changes in labor legislation. At present, general practitioners (on salary) can practice on Saturday mornings and outside regular office hours on a fee-sharing basis. This includes an emergency system with doctors on call.

- *Supporting a sense of ownership among employees:* Trade unions pose a major problem for the delivery of services in the public sector. Low salaries and poor working conditions led to a vicious circle, where both government and trade unions are in a permanent struggle. This struggle usually interferes with any effort to improve the system for the benefit of patients. PROSALUD approached this issue by addressing the needs and demands of employees in an institutionalized way so a trade union became unnecessary. Key interventions are participation of employees in decision-making, transparency in finances, adherence to labor laws, and good working conditions. The sense of ownership achieved was vital to promoting the idea that a trade union was not necessary to meet most of the employees' reasonable expectations. Furthermore, in 1997, the PROSALUD Club was created for social, cultural, and sports events. This activity is financed with voluntary employee contributions and managed independently.

Staffing Patterns

PROSALUD's staff is its main asset, and the organization's personnel recruitment criteria, process, and procedures are crucial elements of the PROSALUD model. The recruitment system is designed to ensure that employees are well qualified and that they share the organization's philosophy and public service goals. Training opportunities, orientation sessions for new staff, and regular staff meetings transmit the

Table 2. PROSALUD Basic Staffing Pattern

Position	Basis of Compensation	No. at Basic Clinic
Medical director*	Salaried general practitioner	1
Specialists* (Ob/Gyn and pediatrician)	Part-time, paid on fee-sharing basis	2
Registered nurse	Salaried	1
Nurse midwife	Salaried (24-hour coverage)	3
Nurse's aide	Salaried (24-hour coverage)	3
Receptionist	Salaried	1
Laboratory technician	Salaried/shared among clinics	1
Community health worker	Salaried	1
Cleaning staff	Salaried	1

*These physicians share responsibility for providing emergency care 24 hours a day at all clinics. A minimum of one doctor is on call at all times. Ambulance and nursing staff are also available 24 hours a day.

Note: The basic clinic serves a catchment area of approximately 15,000, and its workload for curative care averages 13,000 to 15,000 visits per year.

organization's values and culture. A positive environment for employee motivation, commitment, and performance is one of the priorities of the management.

Personnel costs represent two-thirds of total network costs. To improve efficiency and minimize fixed costs, PROSALUD personnel work under two schemes: on salary and on a fee-sharing basis. Table 2 presents the basic clinic staffing pattern.

Clinics provide consultation rooms, ancillary medical services, and support staff to general practitioners (on salary and one per clinic) and specialists (on a fee-sharing basis). PROSALUD provides marketing, management, and clerical support. The Management Support Unit helps to bring in new patients through marketing, promotions, and referrals within the clinics. Support includes bookkeeping and other services, such as receptionist, pharmacist, nursing staff, laboratory services, clerical services, and maintenance. Training opportunities are also provided. In return for these services, the specialists split the fees generated from services provided (the splitting arrangement is determined according to market demand and other factors). In order to operate in the clinic, practitioners are required to abide by PROSALUD's quality standards and procedures.

Table 3. Total PROSALUD Staffing (as of March 1999)

Position	Number
Operational (clinics and referral hospitals)	
Doctors*	162
Dentists†	27
Pharmacists	5
Registered nurses	39
Nurse's aides	107
Laboratory technicians	23
Health promoters	17
Administrative staff (receptionists)	50
Support personnel (drivers, maintenance, etc.)	49
Administrative (HQ and regional offices)	
Executives	13
Middle managers	27
Administrative staff	29
Support personnel	35
TOTAL	583

*72% on fee-sharing arrangements
†100% on fee-sharing arrangements

Clinic staff members operate as a team. Each month, every PRO-SALUD facility reviews its plan for addressing management quality, training, and marketing. All staff members discuss achievements and the difficulties encountered during the development of these activities and how they plan to address these problems in the short term. A combination of self-evaluation and peer evaluation is used in an informal and constructive forum.

Table 3 shows the composition of PROSALUD's staff, including the staff of the social marketing program.

Community Involvement

PROSALUD aims to increase the delivery of essential health services and information at the community level. Each PROSALUD clinic is staffed with community health workers, who promote services, supply family planning commodities, arrange for health education, and follow up with clients to ensure that appropriate treatment has been provided. To bolster the accessibility of services and ties with the local community, each PROSALUD clinic includes a conference room for public use.

A community advisory committee composed of community members and PROSALUD staff oversees each clinic. These committees continuously interact with community members to evaluate local satisfaction with PROSALUD services. Committees are responsible for making recommendations to the clinic management representing client and community needs.

Input from community members regarding PROSALUD services is sought through the following channels:

- cooperation with women's and youth groups
- qualitative (focus groups and in-depth interviews) and quantitative research (marketing surveys, client satisfaction surveys) to determine community health needs and demands and evaluate client satisfaction
- interaction between PROSALUD medical staff, community health workers, clients, and members of the community.

Marketing of Services

PROSALUD uses social marketing techniques to promote its services and products to the public at the network level. PROSALUD markets itself using its appealing brand name and logo, representing high-quality, affordable health care. The PROSALUD logo, services, and products are marketed using a variety of mass media, such as television, radio, billboards, stickers, posters, and health fairs and other community events.

PROSALUD also manages a national reproductive health social marketing project, with assistance from Population Services International (PSI). Since 1995, PSI and PROSALUD have collaborated in promoting and distributing many products, including one female and two male condom brands, three oral contraceptive brands, a water-based lubricant, and an injectable contraceptive. All PROSALUD clinics act as outlets for socially marketed products, and mobile video units of this program advertise PROSALUD services. One of the roles of the community health worker is to promote services and products at the clinic level.

PROSALUD staff members collaborate with other local organizations to develop and conduct large-scale IEC (information, education, and communication) campaigns, using effective social marketing techniques, to raise the public's awareness of the importance of preventive care and thus to generate demand for these priority services. This serves not only to increase demand for services at PROSALUD clinics but also at other private and public facilities.

PROSALUD's staff develops a marketing plan each year. The marketing plan engages the participation of PROSALUD staff and customers in planning and eliciting information about the needs, preferences, and reactions of clients. The plan emphasizes those activities most related to the needs of the population.

Increasing Utilization

PROSALUD attempts to provide not only the curative care demanded by users, but also preventive care that the patient may or may not be managing adequately. PROSALUD has been successful with various forms of promotion, including

- *word of mouth:* Providing high-quality care at a competitive price has proven to be one of the most cost-effective forms of promotion. The majority of patients who come to PROSALUD have heard about it from other satisfied clients. Even when no other techniques have been used, patient volume has increased over time in PROSALUD clinics.

- *health fairs:* Organizing health fairs at each of the clinics, with community participation, has proven to be a very effective and inexpensive form of promotion and advertising. The majority of these fairs combine health education and educational entertainment. They include posters, measuring heights and weights, and a cooking competition to see which mothers' club can prepare the best-tasting meal using the soybeans PROSALUD sells in its pharmacies. In addition, vaccinations are sometimes made available. The immediate impact of these health fairs has been impressive. Some have resulted in a 20% increase in patient volume. Although this increase in volume tends to level out over time, the increased volume usually pays for the health fair several times over and results in several new patients for the centers in the long run—not to mention the indirect benefit of providing health education to the public.

- *mass media:* Radio advertising is the preferred mass medium for PROSALUD, which advertises its services through jingles and health education messages on popular radio stations. TV campaigns for reproductive health and family planning have had good results in raising public awareness about these issues. Television has also been used to promote the institution's image, but it did not have a significant impact on demand.

5
Economic Aspects of PROSALUD

Good health has no price but it always has a cost.
—PROSALUD training materials

This chapter presents PROSALUD's financial model and financial management systems and then discusses how it has applied market principles, for example, in conducting studies of potential sites for new clinics. The chapter concludes with an analysis of PROSALUD's long-term financial sustainability, focusing on the endowment fund.

Financial Model

A system of cross-subsidization among services, units, and clients has been essential to PROSALUD's ability to provide underserved, low-income communities with access to health services. Pricing, fee collection, and provider payment are the components of the financial model that enables PROSALUD to meet this objective.

Pricing
Determining the prices of the services is an important strategy for financial sustainability. In PROSALUD clinics prices vary by geographical area and by type of service. The prices of services are established by considering

- unit costs, factoring in fixed and variable costs
- prices of equivalent services from other providers in the area
- an estimation of the paying capacity of clients

45

- the value of the services to the community
- the opinions of PROSALUD's clinic staff members

The prices of the curative services provided by PROSALUD are slightly higher than those charged at Ministry of Health facilities, but much lower than those at private clinics. The trend has been to price a complete package of services for an episode of illness rather than set prices for individual services. The price of a physician visit, for example, includes the follow-up visit as well as the initial consultation. It does not, however, include medications or laboratory exams.

PROSALUD staff had to make an important management, patient care, and marketing decision in considering what the price includes. By covering both the initial visit and one follow-up visit for the same fee, PROSALUD becomes more competitive with other private institutions. More important, however, is that this kind of fee encourages patients who need a follow-up visit and would not normally see the importance of coming back to the clinic. The exit interview by the nurse is another means of ensuring quality of care, since it reinforces patients' understanding of their medical problem and treatment protocol.

From a medical perspective, diagnostic tests and drugs should be included in the price, since the patient has the best chance of receiving high-quality care if everything is provided under one fee. (If tests and drugs are priced separately, patients may choose not to purchase them.) From a medical management perspective, however, including these services in the fee would probably encourage physicians to request more exams and prescribe more medications than necessary. Charging for these ancillary services motivates physicians to analyze carefully whether the tests and medications are truly needed.

From a marketing perspective, it was determined that including all these services in one fee would require increasing the price of the service to a level that would not be competitive. When a large proportion of the patients have low incomes and levels of education, they are unlikely to be able to compare a fee that includes just the physician visit and one that includes medications, laboratory examinations, and follow-up visits— and perhaps more important, they are not going to have the money to use the health center. A significant number of the poorer patients can afford the initial charge but need to buy their medications a little at a time.

Some patients are truly unable to pay for the services needed. The receptionist who handles the collection of fees determines a patient's ability to pay, in conjunction with the head nurse at the health center. They work out with the patient when possible a means to pay for the service; it might mean that the patient pays something at the time of service and some later.

There was concern that by not using a sliding scale, the nurse and receptionist would make arbitrary decisions about who was to pay and who received free services. This concern has not been warranted for a variety of reasons. First, the decision to provide free services is made by at least two people. (See chapter 8 for more discussion of exemptions and staff training in their application.) In addition, the number of visits and the associated revenues generated are closely monitored at all levels of the organization. It would take only a month to notice that patient visits were not generating the revenues projected, and the medical and nursing supervisors, with the accounting department, would be questioning the staff to ensure that the free services provided were appropriate. A third safeguard against "giving away the store" is that all the staff are aware that their salaries are related to revenues and thus to user fees as well as the quantity of services delivered (demand). The staff becomes adroit in marketing the image of the health center to the community as a health center that accepts all patients, yet the staff also charges for services whenever it is appropriate.

Table 4 provides an illustrative sample of 1998 prices at PROSALUD clinics. There are no fees for preventive services. To keep fees low for curative services, a creative mechanism has been instituted: dividing the fees of specialist services between the clinic and the physician. For those who cannot afford the services, PROSALUD continues to provide nearly 10% of its chargeable services at no cost.

Forms of Payment

Initially, it was difficult to make decisions on pricing and the best means for collecting fees. The concern was whether the community would perceive PROSALUD's services as worth the price. To address this concern, PROSALUD attempted to establish both *fee-for-service* and *prepayment systems*. Since all visits and medications were free under the prepayment system, the result was overutilization and tremendously high drug costs. That program had to be terminated after one year.

PROSALUD soon dropped the prepayment system due to a number of difficulties. However, PROSALUD learned several important lessons from this exploration of the use of a prepaid scheme. First, they learned

Table 4. PROSALUD Fee Schedule (1998)

Service	Range of Fees	
	Local Currency	US$
General medical visit	15–20	2.72–3.63
Specialist visit	20–30	3.63–5.44
Complete blood count	15–20	2.72–3.63
IUD insertion (includes the IUD)	25	4.54
Pap smear	18	3.27
Pregnancy test	15–20	2.72–3.63
Urinalysis	12–15	2.18–2.72
Deliveries	120–150	21.78–27.22
Injections (includes the syringe)	4–5	0.73–0.91

Note: US$1 = Bolivianos (Bs.) 5.51. This was the average 1998 exchange rate, per the Instituto Nacional de Estadística, Bolivia.

that complete cost information is required for setting premiums. Second, they learned that it was imperative to educate clients about how prepaid schemes spread risk among enrolled community members and are not individual "savings accounts." Patients also need to understand why premiums are collected on a regular basis rather than only when service is desired, as in a fee-for-service system. PROSALUD also realized that it was necessary to create incentives for the enrollees in the system in order to control utilization and the costs of the enrolled population through mechanisms such as prepayment. Finally, PROSALUD learned that a prepayment system requires significant market penetration so that there is an adequate base to spread the risk and to ensure that there is not adverse selection.

Based on this experience, PROSALUD established a fee-for-service structure designed to be competitively priced with private health clinics, charging separate fees for consultations, laboratory tests, and drugs. The goal was to provide high-quality services at reasonable prices, resulting in a high volume of services. This form of payment represents 95% of all revenues.

As a result of a health care needs assessment in the industrial area of Santa Cruz City, PROSALUD offered companies a *deferred payment plan* that consists of enrolling employees in their system and billing the companies at the end of each month for the services provided. It guaranteed that employees would be seen on the day they appeared for services; the government Social Security health services frequently had long waiting times for outpatient services. Some firms enrolled in the PROSALUD program, even though by law they still had to pay mandatory Social Security contributions for each employee. Their willingness to pay twice for employees' health care reflected their confidence that PROSALUD would provide fast, high-quality service, enabling employees to return to work more quickly than if they depended on the Social Security system to solve health problems. This form of payment represents 5% of total user fees. The potential of this form of payment is limited by current legislation.

Provider Payment Incentives

PROSALUD's management foresaw that it would be difficult to convince general practitioners to work for four hours on Saturday mornings because other health centers and doctors' offices were not open during this time. However, they felt that the communities' members strongly favored having access to services outside normal working hours. PROSALUD therefore took the risk of offering these doctors a considerably higher portion of the patient revenues generated on Saturdays than they could earn on weekdays. One expected result of this change was that there was a high proportion of working people, particularly men, who came to the clinics on Saturdays. A significant portion of the patients coming to the health center on Saturdays were also first-time patients, that is, those who had not previously received their care at PROSALUD.

PROSALUD applied the risk-sharing incentive system in a different manner for specialists. A fee per visit was established for physician specialty services, and this was divided 50/50 between PROSALUD and the physician. This system was important for two reasons. First, PROSALUD's risk in offering these additional specialties was reduced because physicians had an incentive to "bring in" additional patients to PROSALUD, to increase their personal income. At the same time the overall demand for patient services was increased. This happened because wives (and children) who might ordinarily go to another health center were more willing to come to centers that could also provide their husbands with care and vice versa.

If PROSALUD and the physicians had shared the marginal costs of the specialty clinics, physicians would have been deterred from participating because they and PROSALUD would be equally at risk if few patients came to the specialty clinics. Although the overall reimbursement to the physicians might have been greater in the event of a large patient volume, PROSALUD's executives decided that it was unlikely that they could attract physicians under this arrangement. The fact was that these specialty clinics often generate little to no overall surplus, and more often than not serve as the "loss leaders" to attract the other family members to the health centers.

The Financial Implications of Adding a Health Center

The decision to add a health center to the PROSALUD system is delicate and must be based on a global analysis of the situation inside and outside PROSALUD, since it has both financial and social implications. It was essential to take into account the financial impact of starting a new center: will it generate a financial surplus or incur a deficit? The self-financing of PROSALUD depends on the balance of the financial results of all health centers. Some health centers generate a surplus, others break even, and others incur deficits. The balance enables PROSALUD to provide a percentage of free care by "cross-subsidizing" centers that run a deficit with those that generate a surplus. For example, services in lightly populated rural areas may be financially deficient, but the social impact of serving them may warrant their inclusion in the PROSALUD network.

Financial Management Systems

From the beginning, the financial and management information systems evolved to support the organization's structures. The financial and accounting systems were created to support management decisions at all levels—the central Board of Directors, the Assembly of Associates, and the Director, staff, and community members at each clinic. The computerized accounting system that was developed integrated both financial and patient care statistics. In addition, each clinic was set up as an individual cost center, so that the financial status of each health center is calculated every month. The health center staff and the medical and nursing supervisors review the monthly financial status of the clinic.

Accounting reports are available in two levels of detail. The one used by the health center staff includes the sources of patient revenues and related activities (for example, physician and nurse visits, laboratory tests, and dental visits). The staff receives a breakdown of expenses, which consolidates personnel costs and provides line item information for other operational costs, such as supplies, marketing, maintenance, and percentage contribution to overhead.

These health center budgets are the result of a "costing out" of the activities clinics agreed to perform for the coming year. The director of finance is responsible for developing the budget with information from clinic staff and for having it preliminarily approved at the central level. Then the health center staff review this budget so they fully understand the financial implications of their decisions. Once agreed upon and approved, the budget is broken down by quarter, and progress monitored every month.

The annual work plan is basically a budget constructed to assist these individuals with monitoring activities and tracking income and expenses. The work plan gives an overview of every major activity conducted at the clinic. The provider activities that generated income in the past year are shown, with the number of services provided and the revenues from each type of activity. The clinic director and staff, for example, can immediately see exactly how many services each type of provider performed each month and the number of associated ancillary services. With this detail, they can compare these actual activities with those projected to see if they are on track financially and begin to assess the patient care provided. For example, this information has made it possible to look at the ratios of physician consults to laboratory tests performed and medications provided. It is also possible to evaluate whether clinicians are using an appropriate amount of supplies to care for patients.

Clinics' budgets include some funds for training, marketing, and maintenance. Although the bulk of these services are provided centrally to take advantage of economies of scale, PROSALUD's executives felt that each clinic should have some funds available for these services so they could respond to the health center needs efficiently. For example, if they needed to make minor repairs, they did not have to wait for approval and someone to come from the central level to do something as simple and immediate as repair a light fixture. Or if they decided that they wanted to hold a health care fair for the community, they would have funds to do this.

Understanding Market Dynamics

An understanding and application of basic market principles, such as supply and demand and the promotion of services, has been important to PROSALUD's success. During the planning, organization, and management of the organization's cost-recovery strategy, the analysis of market dynamics was consistently used as a managerial tool. Using a market analysis approach in decision-making included conducting studies to study the relationships between supply and demand, as well as the market's relationship to morbidity and mortality trends ("felt needs" of consumers versus "unfelt needs"). PROSALUD also uses techniques that increase demand at clinics, while taking time and money constraints into account.

Market Research
The opening of new health centers is determined based on market studies that project unmet and potential demand, community income levels, staffing needs, mix of services, the cost of services to be provided, and competition. After some trials, PROSALUD developed an efficient methodology for assessing the potential for locating a PROSALUD facility in a community.

Determining the feasibility of starting a new clinic through a market study. The first step in determining whether a clinic will be located in a particular area is to conduct a market study to evaluate the characteristics of the market and potential demand. These characteristics inform decision-makers about the feasibility of locating a health care center in a given area.

The market study uses a census that identifies the characteristics, needs, and demands of the population. This is not a survey but an actual census, because many of the rural and periurban areas do not have addresses or any reliable source of information. Therefore, every house is covered in the census—often up to 3,000 families. The geographic area in question is circumscribed before conducting the census, which PROSALUD staff members carry out with the help of trained community personnel.

The census form is easy to use and includes the following information:

- address
- number of occupants
- length of time in the area
- family structure
- ethnic group
- mother's and father's occupation, place of employment, and level of education
- health insurance affiliation and degree of satisfaction with health insurance
- preference of health care providers
- morbidity over the past two weeks
- predisposition to pay for health care services and under which conditions.

This marketing study does not attempt to collect statistically significant data for use in a sophisticated econometric study analyzing key factors that influence demand. It is a study to help managers to determine whether it is feasible and socially desirable to place a health center in a designated area, and, if so, what the community's capacity to sustain this service financially will be.

Like most small institutions, PROSALUD does not have the resources or the time to conduct lengthy and extensive studies. Often a potential donor does not wish to wait a year for PROSALUD to respond about where they could best use funding. They need to provide answers for donors within months. The questions asked of community members are therefore limited in number and scope, and the data do not necessarily represent a full picture of the health care demand patterns of a given community. The questions in the census are also simple enough for minimally trained collectors to use and simple enough to allow rapid tabulation after the data are collected.

The data from this study are used in evaluating the feasibility of a health care center and in defining and planning its services. For operational and financial planning, the market studies have proven to be highly reliable. Data from these studies are the basis of work plans and help managers to set goals for volume of activities by service.

Determining the best means of meeting people's needs and demands through studies of the health care market. Once the decision is made to establish a clinic in a certain area, the preliminary data, and sometimes subsequent studies, are used to further analyze the dynamics among demand, needs, and supply. With this information, implementation and marketing plans are developed that define locations, objectives, methods for measuring impact, budgets, and promotion and advertising strategies and tactics.

Long-Term Sustainability: The Endowment Fund

Over the years, PROSALUD has matured into a sophisticated organization, serving as a model for new and cost-effective modes of service delivery, while balancing two distinct objectives: serving low-income populations with high-quality health services while pursing financial sustainability. To date, PROSALUD has demonstrated a considerable degree of financial sustainability from cost recovery, particularly in the mature centers, but has yet to achieve full self-sustainability.

PROSALUD recently carried out a long-term financial planning process and identified and began implementing strategies that will eventually lead to financial self-sustainability (Holley 1996). This plan, however, in the absence of additional sources of income, clearly demonstrates the necessity of raising prices slightly in order to reach the break-even point. Unfortunately, such action would have the inevitable effect of excluding a portion of PROSALUD's existing clientele in favor of a more middle-class population and work directly against PROSALUD's other strategies for achieving financial sustainability, which are based on increasing demand and volume of services rather than prices. See Figure 5, "PROSALUD Model for Analyzing the Financial Sustainability of a Health Care System."

This model begins with the determination of the catchment population (number of people and their basic demographic characteristics) of a clinic or clinic network. The next step is the analysis of their *needs* and *demands*, which defines probable felt needs, unfelt needs, and unnecessary demands of the population. The result of the analysis, which takes demographic, epidemiological, and market data into account, is a definition of the *supply* of the system, that is, the package of health care services.

Figure 5. PROSALUD Model for Analyzing the Financial Sustainability of a Health Care System

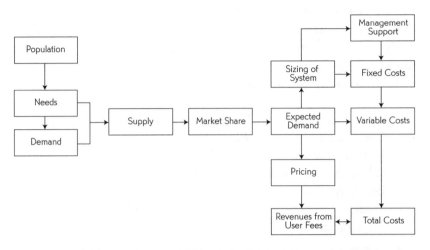

With the data from the market survey, the *market share* of a clinic or clinic network in a given situation is estimated. With the information on needs, demand, supply, and market share, it is possible to calculate *expected demand* by type of service. Expected demand, as Figure 5 shows, affects the *sizing of the system, variable costs*, and *pricing*. These factors in turn influence the *management support* required and the *fixed costs*. The model concludes by analyzing the *total costs* of the clinic or clinic network compared to the *revenues from user fees*. In PROSALUD's experience, the application of this model permits a better understanding of market dynamics, and it has become an essential tool for decision-making.

The purpose, therefore, of the endowment that PROSALUD received from the US Agency for International Development in September 1997 is to provide the additional income PROSALUD requires to achieve financial self-sustainability while maintaining prices that lower-income people can afford. PROSALUD requested an initial $2 million from USAID in 1997, with an additional $1 million per year from 1998 to 2000, for a total of $5 million (of which it has received $4 million to date).

PROSALUD is in a period of expansion, supported by USAID. Between 1996 and the end of 1999, PROSALUD opened eight new clinics and expanded services in existing ones. These centers will achieve maturity and economic self-sufficiency in the early years of the new century.

Purpose and Objectives of the Endowment

The purpose of the endowment is to help PROSALUD to become an independent, financially self-sustaining organization that can indefinitely provide and continue to expand high-quality primary health care services to poor and lower-middle-class Bolivians at reasonable prices. The three objectives of the endowment are to

- finalize the creation of PROSALUD as an independent organization and ensure that it will continue its mission in the absence of further external funding. PROSALUD has had, and thus will be able to continue to have, an impact on the entire Bolivian primary health care system. Furthermore, it will continue to serve as a model and prototype for the establishment of similar systems throughout the world.

- permit PROSALUD to establish policies and implement strategies that will lead to financial self-sufficiency, while not sacrificing its commitment to serve low-income populations. Additional support is required to allow PROSALUD the time necessary to reach its maximum capacity in terms of services and coverage. Short-term grants will not provide PROSALUD with the financial stability to carry out significant long-term policy changes.

- enable PROSALUD not only to continue to provide curative health services to low-income populations, but also to allow it to continue to provide a wide variety of preventive and public health services. The latter include reproductive health services, including sex education, family planning, and AIDS prevention.

Growth of the Endowment Fund

The endowment fund has three basic sources of income:

- seed capital ($5 million) from USAID

- surplus, if any, from operations, estimated at $1.5 million for 1996 and 1997

- interest income, which is projected at more than $400,000 per year after the first few years.

With the initial endowment contributions of $5 million through 2000 and any surplus balances contributed by PROSALUD operations, it is projected that the endowment balance will grow from $1.9 million in 1998 to over $7.5 million by 2007. These projections assume a conservative 6% return on the endowment fund balance and a decrease in the cost of managing the endowment fund from 1.5% of the value of the endowment in 1998 to 1.0% in 2007.

The ultimate purpose of the endowment is to help PROSALUD to reach the financial break-even point. If by adding endowment income to its operational income, PROSALUD is able to completely cover its operational expenses, the endowment will have served its purpose. (See the conclusion for details about the government's contribution to services for the poor.)

In the medium term, PROSALUD will withdraw some of the income from the fund to cover operating expenses. This is considered legitimate as long as the withdrawals are neither excessive nor prolonged. The endowment is meant to supplement PROSALUD's operational income, not replace it, and in fact, the endowment income in the year 2006 is projected to represent only about 6% of total income. That 6%, however, is the margin required to continue providing high-quality services to low-income populations without raising prices above the rate of inflation. This endowment fund will provide a solid financial base for securing the future growth of PROSALUD.

Management of the Endowment
The endowment is managed by the Endowment Committee of the Board of Directors, which contracted a professional asset manager based in the United States. The investment policy of the endowment is to secure a reasonable rate of return while minimizing risk. USAID will approve all disbursements during the life of the endowment agreement and monitor closely the progress of PROSALUD in its efforts to achieve financial self-sustainability, as well as the management of the endowment fund itself.

Achieving Financial Independence
In addition to the financial support provided by USAID, PROSALUD is pursuing an ambitious program of reengineering in order to achieve financial independence. Its mission and objectives, as well as the basic model of health care provision, remain the same, but to reach financial

independence, the organization is tightening its management and adapting its organizational perspective and behavior to new challenges and opportunities. PROSALUD has already embarked on a program designed to achieve these results (Holley 1996). It includes, among other measures, activities to obtain contributions from other donors for the endowment fund.

6
Achievements of PROSALUD

PROSALUD has developed a model for providing essential public health services as well as desired private health services to underserved populations. The model ensures that the services provided are of high quality clinically while maintaining reasonable and affordable prices. This chapter details its major achievements:

- expanding coverage
- stressing financial sustainability through efficient operations and cost recovery
- working with the public sector
- raising quality standards
- contributing to health sector reform in Bolivia.

Extending Coverage and the Range of Services to Communities

In Bolivia PROSALUD is the single largest nongovernmental organization in the health field. As of the end of 1999, PROSALUD's network of health services serves a population of 500,000, which represents approximately 13% of the urban population of Bolivia. PROSALUD clinics have a market share of 20% in the urban areas they serve.

PROSALUD has gained considerable experience in providing efficient, cost-effective health care. It has developed a full range of treatment protocols and clinical procedures and has a strong reputation for responding to community needs. The basic delivery model it developed has proven successful in a variety of environments. This model

Figure 6. Growth of the Number of PROSALUD Health Services Provided per Year

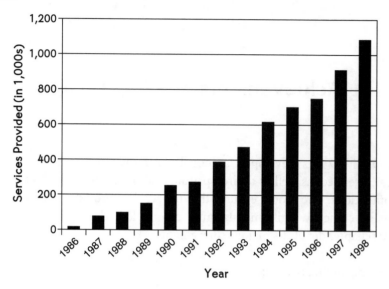

continues to evolve, as PROSALUD seeks to refine its staffing patterns to achieve greater cost-effectiveness.

The total number of health services provided by PROSALUD has risen for 13 consecutive years, to over one million in 1998 (see Figure 6). These services cover a wide range, including medical and nursing care, deliveries, well-baby and antenatal clinics, immunizations, laboratory and radiology services, and home care visits. The balance of services is evidenced by the mix of services delivered: preventive services account for 34% of all services provided, while curative and ancillary services each account for another third. These data illustrate that PROSALUD is providing services to meet community needs rather than focusing on the most profitable services, such as curative care.

Integrating Family Planning Services into the PROSALUD Delivery System

In 1989, the government incorporated family planning services into the national mother and child health program. This health policy allows PROSALUD and other organizations to provide family planning services in response to unmet demand. Figure 7 shows the evolution of the number of new family planning users since this program was integrated into PROSALUD activities. The integration of the family planning program

Figure 7. Growth of the Number of New Family Planning Users

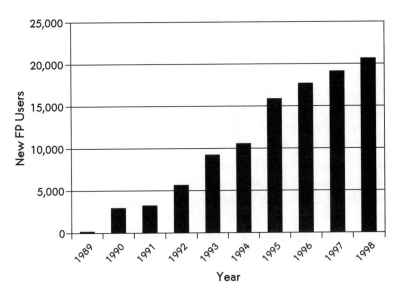

Note: Family planning became part of the MOH programs in late 1989.

was designed to preserve its identity in the delivery system while using the capacity of all clinics. All clinics provide family planning services, at the same time as other services, and virtually all personnel are involved. Integration prevented having to hire additional staff and enhanced the ability of all personnel to respond to demand with high-quality services.

Financial and Operational Sustainability

PROSALUD has managed to achieve a remarkable record in terms of cost recovery despite its commitment to serve low-income populations with high-quality services. The clinics in Santa Cruz recovered 83.6% of their total costs in 1997; in La Paz and El Alto, which is a newer network serving a poorer population, the figure reached 60.1%. In Tarija and Riberalta (which have both operated for less than two years), cost recovery has reached 51.6% and 83.6%, respectively. The overall cost recovery rate is 70.9%.

The difference has been covered by other sources of income and support from USAID as part of the plan to reach financial self-sufficiency.

The challenge for the future is to continue providing more and better services to low-income populations while achieving full financial self-sustainability supported by the endowment fund.

The challenge of financial sustainability is illustrated in the figures in Table 5. Note the difference in cost-recovery rates among different facilities. This shows how self-sufficiency among a network of clinics is more easily attained than in just one facility, since each serves different communities. The advantage of the network structure is greater risk sharing and the possibility of cross-subsidies. The figures also show clearly that even with positive cost-recovery rates in providing health services, the costs of management can impede financial self-sufficiency. It is crucial to financial sustainability to have efficient management at minimal cost, to reduce the burden of administrative expenses on clinics.

A USAID-funded study conducted by University Research Corporation and the International Science and Technology Institute (Richardson et al. 1992) focused on two Ministry of Health and two PROSALUD health centers and looked at quality, costs, and cost recovery. The findings revealed that the volumes of services delivered by the MOH and by PROSALUD were significantly different. Coverage of the target population of MOH facilities was low, as measured by per capita curative visits per year: the MOH averaged 0.24, while PROSALUD averaged 0.97. The report mentioned that there is no reason to expect that size, socioeconomic status, or service characteristics affected the production of services.

The URC/ISTI study findings about PROSALUD's sustainability were that

- PROSALUD's unit costs were lower than those of MOH clinics
- PROSALUD staff were more productive than MOH staff in terms of services rendered per provider
- cost-recovery percentages were higher in PROSALUD facilities than in MOH facilities
- PROSALUD's catchment population made greater use of services (nearly 1 visit per person per year for PROSALUD members compared to .25 visits per year at MOH facilities)
- PROSALUD facilities were more efficient in their operations than MOH facilities.

The efficiency with which the health centers operate is directly

Table 5. Operating Revenues and Expenses of the PROSALUD Network (1997)

	Revenues	Expenses	Operating Surplus (Deficit)	Cost Recovery of Services Provided (%)
PROSALUD/Santa Cruz				
Network of services	1,110,091	1,073,676	36,415	103.4
Regional Office		254,641		
Total	*1,110,091*	*1,328,317*	*(218,226)*	*83.6*
PROSALUD/La Paz–El Alto				
Network of services	672,152	915,613	(243,461)	73.4
Regional Office		203,520		
Total	*672,152*	*1,119,133*	*(446,981)*	*60.1*
PROSALUD/Tarija				
Network of services	160,654	208,151	(47,497)	77.2
Regional Office		103,452		
Total	*160,654*	*311,603*	*(150,949)*	*51.6*
PROSALUD/Riberalta				
1 polyclinic	90,221	107,879	(17,658)	83.6
Total	*90,221*	*107,879*	*(17,658)*	*83.6*
GRAND TOTAL	2,033,118	2,866,932	(833,814)	70.9

Notes: Depreciation is included.
Figures are in US$.

related to the sustainability of PROSALUD. In 1992, MOH centers averaged 351 services per provider (physician or nurse), while PROSALUD centers averaged 1,024 services per provider (Richardson et al. 1992). This is critical for accounting for the low level of efficiency in the MOH centers and the high unit costs of service. The low utilization of services in MOH facilities translates into high unit costs for most comparable services. Unit costs average Bs. 4.87 for PROSALUD facilities and Bs. 7.39 in MOH facilities. The PROSALUD unit costs average 66% of the MOH unit costs. Table 6 summarizes these findings.

Strengthening the Private Sector

PROSALUD's positive effects on the private health sector as a whole include

- *linkages with the public sector:* PROSALUD provides a mechanism for linking the private sector with the public sector. In addition to increasing private-sector participation in providing the essential package of services and in various public health campaigns, PRO-SALUD systematically collects and shares statistics with the MOH's Health Information System.

- *job creation:* The PROSALUD network has employed more than 500 people. These jobs include clinical, clerical, and other kinds of employment. Specialists and dentists enjoy the opportunity of working as independent providers and can complement the revenues from their private practices.

- *training:* The PROSALUD network's training efforts have contributed significantly to improve the overall quality of health care in Bolivia. PROSALUD not only trains its own employees but also makes its training facilities available to other medical practitioners. This training provides practitioners with opportunities to hone their skills in both medical services and clinic management.

- *increased capacity:* PROSALUD makes its pharmacy and laboratory services available to other practitioners in Bolivia to improve their ability to provide comprehensive health services. Furthermore, the hospital and polyclinics serve as referral facilities for patients from non-PROSALUD clinics.

Table 6. Health Center Efficiency

Categories	Indicators	MOH Clinics		PROSALUD Clinics	
		V. de Cotoca	Santa Rosita	La Madre	El Carmen
Population	Catchment area	11,800	21,606	8,712	15,243
Staff	Total staff	10	17	10	10
	No. of care providers (FTE)*	7.5	7.0	6.3	7.0
Services	No. of services rendered	1,753	3,330	5,694	7,920
	Services rendered per provider	234	476	904	1,131
	No. of community visits	68	56	224	197
Costs	Total costs	11,393	27,534	29,274	36,461
	Unit cost per service	6.50	8.27	5.14	4.60
	Unit cost per consult	9.67	7.76	7.01	4.10
	Unit cost per birth	110.13	427.19	97.68	90.68
	Unit cost per vaccination	1.42	2.18	1.14	1.49
	Supervision as % of costs	5	2.2	2.9	2.5
Revenues	Fees collected	4,393	18,652	23,965	35,094
	Cost recovery as % of costs	39	68	82	96
	Curative visits per capita per year	0.22	0.26	0.97	0.97

*FTE = full-time equivalent
Note: Costs are in Bolivianos. Rate US$1 = Bs. 3.81.
Source: Adapted from Richardson et al. 1992

- *halo effect:* The franchise network has created competitive pressures that have increased quality among public and private practitioners and clinics and have reduced prices in the private sector in some instances.

Raising Quality Standards

In 1992, the Santa Cruz Regional Health Office requested assistance from the US Agency for International Development's mission in Bolivia to better understand the strengths and weaknesses of its primary health care delivery system in Santa Cruz City and to make recommendations for improving the system and ultimately the health care services provided to MOH clients. The Regional Health Office was concerned about the health needs of the indigent and its ability to provide quality services to this target population.

To identify specific problems and possible solutions, the Regional Health Office suggested that the study analyze the strengths and weaknesses of both the MOH health care system and the PROSALUD system, compare the systems, identify aspects of the PROSALUD system that could be adapted to the MOH system, and recommend alternative solutions compatible with the MOH's scarce resources.

With respect to quality, the URC/ISTI study (Richardson et al. 1992) found that

- the technical quality of direct provider care, as measured by observation, is similar in the two systems (however, critical deficiencies were found in one of the MOH centers)
- patients' perception of quality of care is better in PROSALUD than in MOH facilities
- patient satisfaction with PROSALUD is greater than with the MOH.

Contributing to Health Sector Reform in Bolivia

Over the last 14 years, there have been many changes in both the over-all situation in Bolivia and the health sector. The structural adjust-ments to macroeconomic policies led to dramatic and sudden changes that affected the health sector and, therefore, health institutions and personnel. The mechanisms to cope with this new environment varied according to institutional mandates and vision. Government agencies, nongovernmental organizations, and traditional private-sector providers were forced to emphasize efficiency and short-term results to be consis-tent with the new order. Each designed and implemented different poli-cies, which did not necessarily respond to the health sector reform's long-term objectives.

As an effect of overall structural changes, health sector reform in Bolivia started in 1989. The main characteristics to date include

- further decentralization
- enhanced community involvement
- more action by new public and private entities: municipalities, local governments, nongovernmental organizations, and private providers
- improved targeting of health services
- insurance schemes and subsidies for cost-effective interventions
- increased strategies for sustainability: building the capacity of local organizations, innovative financial mechanisms
- separation of the financial and service provision functions
- changes in the governing function of the MOH.

PROSALUD has helped to meet government goals for the private sector, especially by reducing the burden on the MOH to provide all health services and by improving the overall quality of health care. A PROSALUD-style network is seen as a way to contribute to better organization, greater efficiency, and higher quality of private health services, in particular.

PROSALUD has contributed to health sector reform in Bolivia by

- increasing opportunities and incentives for private providers to deliver essential health services
- expanding access to an affordable package of health interventions through the private sector.

Although PROSALUD was not meant to be a health reform project, it has had a significant impact on both the public and private health sectors in Bolivia. The MOH has adopted several elements of the PRO-SALUD model. In the private commercial sector, the change is even more noticeable. To better compete with PROSALUD's high-quality care at a low cost, prices have fallen and the quality of services has improved. The 1995 external evaluation of PROSALUD (Fiedler and Hougen) identified these indirect effects on the health care market as possibly the most important and enduring effects of the project. In practice, PROSALUD clinics create more competitiveness and make the health market "less imperfect" in the areas in which they operate. These indirect effects are noticeable in both the public and the private sectors and constitute the main practical contributions to health sector reform in Bolivia.

The impact of PROSALUD on the public sector has been principally indirect. In the periurban areas served by PROSALUD clinics, public clinics have experienced increasing competition and therefore an incentive to improve the quality of their clinics through mechanisms such as risk-sharing with specialists (fee-sharing arrangements), 24-hour medical service, and active social marketing campaigns. The impact on the private health sector, however, has been a direct one, which has resulted in reduction of prices, improved compliance with schedules (that is, doctors are present during office hours), and incentives to serve clients better.

7
Replication of the PROSALUD Model in Bolivia

The PROSALUD model has been implemented through a three-step process:

- the establishment of a public-private partnership
- the development of a structure to ensure sustainability and equity
- the development and implementation of management and community involvement techniques.

This approach was replicated through a franchising methodology, which is described at the end of this chapter.

The Public-Private Partnership

In the early stages, PROSALUD defined its position in regard to the public sector as follows:

- PROSALUD as a civic organization will contribute to the national health system and therefore to the Ministry of Health and municipalities, by improving access to and the coverage and quality of health care services for communities.
- PROSALUD recognizes the MOH as the governing entity of the health care sector.
- PROSALUD will be accountable to the MOH and municipalities for the use of resources from government agencies, cooperating agencies, and communities.

- PROSALUD will maintain a high standard of health care management that continually seeks ways to sustain and build the ability to offer more and improved services to the community.
- PROSALUD will search for mechanisms that permit the creation of a true coalition among the public sector, communities, and PROSALUD.

Agreements

In practice, PROSALUD established agreements with the MOH (central and regional) and the municipalities. The agreements were based on the following principles:

- PROSALUD will work with the government to avoid duplication of efforts.
- Community members will participate actively and responsibly.
- Costs will be recovered from user fees and other methods to ensure a solid financial base and therefore contribute to the sustainability of services.
- PROSALUD will manage the system autonomously.

Ministry of Health and local government contribution. According to the agreements, the MOH and local governments contributed to the implementation of a PROSALUD clinic by

- lending or constructing buildings and/or donating land for construction
- delegating delivery of health services in a given area (definition based on a market study)
- monitoring and evaluating the performance and quality of the services
- providing supplies such as vaccines, TB drugs, and malaria drugs for priority programs.

PROSALUD contribution. PROSALUD channeled resources from cooperating agencies and government agencies to

- remodel, improve, or build health facilities

Figure 8. Sources of PROSALUD's 33 Clinics

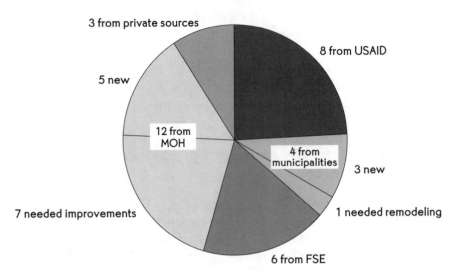

- equip and maintain the clinics
- hire and train personnel according to PROSALUD norms (personnel are not public-sector employees)
- provide administrative and technical support to the clinic network
- ensure quality of services
- follow MOH standards and regulations
- submit statistical and financial information following MOH norms
- ensure community participation.

As a tangible result of this partnership, PROSALUD obtained 30 of its 33 clinics from public-sector sources (only 1 clinic in Riberalta and the hospital in Santa Cruz are owned by PROSALUD). (See Figure 8.) PROSALUD took over 12 clinics from the MOH (5 were new and 7 needed improvements); 6 clinics were funded by the Fondo Social de Emergencia (Social Emergency Fund, a central government agency); municipalities provided 4 clinics (3 were new construction and 1 needed remodeling); and 8 were built with resources from USAID. The municipalities donated the land, reserving the right to take it back if PRO-SALUD failed to comply with the agreement. In 1999 two new clinics were added, in Oruro and Cochabamba cities. Both of them were built with USAID funding on land donated by municipalities.

Guiding Principles: Sustainability and Equity

Sustainability and equity are the guiding principles of PROSALUD. These concepts are defined as follows:

> Sustainability is the institutional capacity to, at least, maintain for the target population in the long term, those health care benefits provided by the project even after the external financing either comes to an end, or is substantially reduced (PROSALUD, "El libro azul," p. 6).

In other words, it is the ability to maintain a positive health impact among target populations over time.

This principle would not be complete without the additional element of equity, which is defined as

> the capacity of the system to provide more services to the community and to respond to their health care needs, taking into account the economic, social, and educational differences and the fact that each individual must contribute in some manner to ensure that the population as a whole reaches not only a better state of health but a higher quality of life (PROSALUD, "El libro azul," p. 6).

Sustainability is a means of ensuring continuity in the delivery of health benefits to the community and not an end in itself. In PRO-SALUD's experience, achieving sustainability requires a process based on the development of three fundamental pillars: institutional development, quality of services, and a solid financial base (see Figure 9).

Institutional Development

The institutional development pillar guarantees the stability of the decision-making elements of the system. This includes three fundamental components:

Figure 9. PROSALUD's Pillars of Sustainability

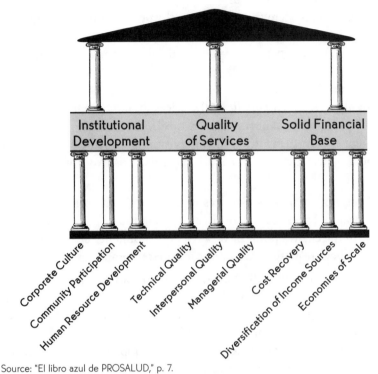

Source: "El libro azul de PROSALUD," p. 7.

- A *corporate culture* was developed that empowers employees and fosters a socially conscious and client-oriented environment. This implies the establishment of corporate bylaws, policies, delivery models, procedures, protocols, and quality standards.

- The establishment of mechanisms for *community participation* entailed the creation of a Board of Directors for the organization and local health committees for each clinic, so that the community recipients of care feel a genuine sense of ownership of the health care centers. Community leaders, organizations, and members have the opportunity to express their needs through focus groups, censuses, and periodic meetings, thus contributing to institutional development.

- The *development of human resources*, as a planned process, is necessary to ensure satisfactory performance, labor stability, and preparedness for the future.

High-Quality Health Services

The creation of a system that guarantees the production of high-quality health services is the second component of sustainability. In the context of PROSALUD, quality is achieved with the development of three components:

- *Technical (medical) quality:* All services should be delivered strictly following medical norms and protocols. This includes the enforcement of standards through supervision and medical audits. The goal of technical quality is to maximize positive impact on the health of the population.

- *Interpersonal quality:* Services must be not only technically good but should also be delivered in a kind way and be perceived as good from the client's point of view. Clients should be satisfied and feel that they are getting good value for their time and resources.

- *Managerial quality:* PROSALUD pays close attention to increasing efficiency in the delivery of its services to ensure that prices remain affordable to the target population. Managerial quality derives from a positive organizational culture, systems that work to produce well-trained staff, appropriately equipped facilities, essential drugs and supplies, and information for decision-making.

Solid Financial Base

The implementation of mechanisms that contribute to maintaining a solid financial base is the third component of sustainability. The development of this component is the goal of self-financing, which is the capacity of the system to generate revenues that come directly from the community, as equitably as possible, so that these revenues constitute the primary source of income for the organization and cover a significant portion of the organization's costs. Once again, self-financing is a critical component, but it is not the only element necessary to become self-sufficient. In PROSALUD's experience, there are three main elements of a solid financial base:

- *Cost recovery with cross-subsidization:* PROSALUD recovers a significant amount of its costs with revenue generated by user fees charged for selected, mostly curative, services. The fee-for-service system creates cross-subsidies at three levels: First, curative services subsidize the provision of preventive care. Second, clinics generating surplus revenues support the operations of those clinics running a deficit. Third, users who can afford to pay subsidize care, to a certain extent, for those who cannot afford to pay.

- *Diversification of sources of income:* In addition to revenues generated from user fees, PROSALUD sells health-related services and products such as contraceptives, eyeglasses, and orthopedic devices. PROSALUD also generates funds through training, research, and technical assistance for other organizations. Finally, the endowment fund was established in 1997 as a complementary source of revenue.

- *Economies of scale:* The PROSALUD network provides a unique opportunity to attain substantial economies of scale to reduce its costs. Economies of scale are being applied mainly through sharing of technical resources among clinics, use of multipurpose personnel, and procurement in bulk for the entire system.

Putting the Model into Practice: Management and "Animation"

The "Management-Animation Model," originally conceived by the Department of Public Health of the Institute of Tropical Medicine in Antwerp, Belgium, illustrates a global approach to health problems in the context of development (see Figure 10). PROSALUD relies on this model to explain its general strategy and to guide its day-to-day activities toward sustainability.

According to the model, the health sector in developing countries faces three major obstacles:

- the existence of significant problems in public health, reflected in high rates of morbidity and mortality
- the scarcity—both quantitative and qualitative—of physical, technological, financial, and human resources, and inadequate distribution
- the fatalistic attitude of many people, especially the poor, which is the product of successive frustrations; this translates into a loss of

Figure 10. Management-Animation Model

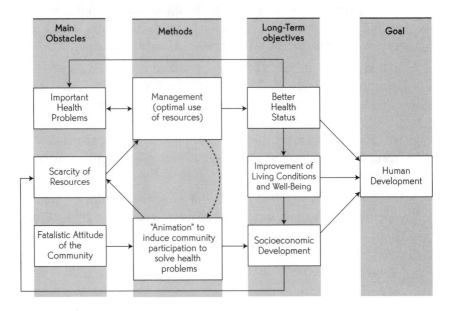

Source: Adapted from Department of Public Health, Institute of Tropical Medicine, International Course in Health Development, Antwerp, Belgium, 1981–82.

faith and self-confidence and into the lack of participation in the solution of common problems.

The response to this situation is a set of management and "animation" (community participation) activities to be used in a timely and integrated manner. In PROSALUD's experience, this model was a very useful tool to communicate with service providers. Both the management and animation activities have become part of the corporate culture.

The animation process aims to motivate community members and induce them to be an active part of the solution of their health problems. Animation activities include community empowerment, establishment of local health committees, training of health promoters, health promotion activities, and home visits.

The community resources generated through user fees are administered in a responsible, efficient, and transparent manner, using modern management principles. PROSALUD defines management as the optimal utilization of community and institutional resources in order to achieve sustainability, which enables the system to maximize health benefits in the population in an equitable fashion.

At the operational level, the main management activities are market analysis, annual work plans, management of information systems, data-based decision-making, quality assurance, franchising, and monitoring and evaluation of financial performance. The combination of management and animation activities has proven essential to put the model into practice at the delivery level.

Franchising

Franchising Concepts and Methodologies

Franchising is a mechanism for replicating a proven business strategy. In the PROSALUD context, franchising principles and methodologies have been applied to support replication of the model in geographically and culturally different cities of Bolivia and to incorporate private providers into PROSALUD clinics on a fee-sharing basis.

In PROSALUD's experience, franchising of health services can

- expedite and facilitate the development of private-sector health care provision
- increase the ability to create and satisfy demand
- reduce the burden on the public sector to provide all health services by private-sector cooperation and competition with the public sector in different spheres of influence.

The franchising concepts and methodologies that PROSALUD uses include

- definition of the business framework
- market and feasibility studies
- definition of locations
- standardization
- corporate image

- quality control
- distinctive supervision style
- decentralized management systems
- marketing and advertising
- incentives for providers and managers
- pricing strategies

Roles of Franchiser and Franchisees

The National Office acts as the "franchiser" and takes charge of defining the business framework, which includes policies, quality standards, norms and protocols, physical requirements (including equipment), and administrative procedures. The National Office is also in charge of all personnel procedures, including recruitment, hiring, and training.

Regional Offices are the "franchisees" and therefore are in charge of establishing all the components of the business framework in their network. In the implementation phase, the franchiser helps the franchisee to build up the delivery system. Once the system is implemented, the franchisee progressively assumes all management functions in a decentralized fashion. The franchiser exercises quality and financial control as well as providing technical assistance and coordinating promotion and marketing activities. The instruments that regulate this relationship are the corporate bylaws and manuals.

The Regional Offices franchise the clinics with private doctors and dentists working on a fee-sharing basis. In this case, the Regional Office becomes the franchiser and the physicians, the franchisees. The Regional Office provides private practitioners with appropriate infrastructure, supplies, and technical and management support. The franchisees are motivated to provide better-quality health care by sharing user fees. An enforceable agreement governs the relationship between both parties.

The next chapter analyzes obstacles that arose as the organization evolved and how it responded. Chapter 9 includes a discussion of what PROSALUD learned about the replication of the model in other cities in Bolivia and presents some of the conditions needed for the PROSALUD experience to be applied in other countries.

8
Major Challenges Addressed
by PROSALUD

The level of development that PROSALUD has reached since 1985 resulted from a long and difficult learning process, and many of its achievements were the product of mistakes and learning from those experiences. PROSALUD has achieved many of the major goals established at its inception. But the road that the organization has traveled has not been easy, and the distance still to go will not be either. The organization will continue to face obstacles and challenges that will test its tenacity and creative capacity. For example, although it has made remarkable achievements in becoming financially sustainable, PROSALUD is not totally self-sufficient financially today.

Due to the problems that surrounded the start-up of PROSALUD, the health care delivery model and the health services management model had to be designed at the same time as they were being implemented. Because of PROSALUD's novelty there were few references to guide the crafting of solutions to the conceptual and operational problems that arose and which are discussed in the following sections.

Market Issues

Learning to Understand the Market
The simultaneous installation of a new economic model in the country was propitious for the implementation of the project, but it also threatened PROSALUD's ability to learn how to conduct itself in a free market economy and in a country where the government fixed prices on the basis of subsidies and political motives. The attempt to understand and

apply this knowledge was a major problem in the first phase of the project. The efforts to plan the first two clinics followed the old model of public planning: planning based on the "needs" of the population, as defined by norms established by the MOH. This focus had negative consequences, since the first PROSALUD clinic in Santa Cruz was designed with an excessive number of personnel in relation to the demand of its catchment area. The result was a low level of cost recovery, an expensive lesson that changed the focus of planning for new clinics thereafter. Planning was no longer based on theoretical needs but on the actual and potential demand for services in a clinic's catchment area.

Another problem was where to locate new clinics. The first ones were located in inappropriate places, taking into account only if the community was receptive or a facility available and not the market and its potential for supporting self-financing services. The market studies that were initially carried out were not related to the decision to open a clinic at a given site. In reality, the study was carried out only after a basically subjective decision to open a clinic had already been made. Therefore, the usefulness of the market studies was very limited, as reflected by low utilization and cost-recovery rates. PROSALUD's managers learned that the decision-making process for opening a clinic at a given site had to include a quantitative evaluation of the market. From this experience, PROSALUD established norms and procedures for the opening of new clinics, using instruments (the census, for example) that had a high predictive value in measuring the potential of the market.

Obtaining the Support of the Community

The maxim that "Good ideas don't sell themselves" was particularly apt when it came to obtaining community support in neighborhoods where PROSALUD intended to expand its services. In theory, one might think that no one could oppose the establishment of a clinic in an underserved area. In practice, in every community there were groups with special interests that might be opposed to the overall interests of the community. In PROSALUD's experience, health personnel resisted the arrival of a "competitor" the most. The active or passive resistance of doctors, nurses, or pharmacists was the principal obstacle to gaining community support in the evaluation phase of the feasibility of a new clinic. Numerous meetings and conversations with community members, backed by the data from the market studies, were essential to overcome this resistance.

Other problems were related to the quality of the leadership of community organizations. Some leaders offered their support in exchange for certain advantages or privileges (such as employment of a family member or free health services). Because PROSALUD staff did not yield to these pressures, occasional resistance and resentment arose.

Community participation also faced the obstacle of prejudices about the "privatization" of the public health sector. This is one reason why some community leaders resisted the idea of having a PROSALUD clinic in their area. Organizing visits by community leaders to existing clinics was one means of counteracting these prejudices, which seemed to arise more from fear of the unknown than from any ideological motive.

Physical Resource Issues

Obtaining Land or Buildings

One practical aspect of the public-private partnership is the use of facilities or the assignment of land, under the system of lease agreements that enable PROSALUD to operate. Obtaining land or buildings was difficult because it was necessary to negotiate their location with local Ministry of Health and municipal officials. Negotiating sites required PROSALUD to confront technical problems (distribution of facilities, target population) and legal problems (property deeds, approval of the city council). At first, conflicts arose with authorities who wanted to impose the location of a clinic in a place that PROSALUD's managers believed would not be convenient for clients or viable in terms of the market.

For all these reasons, PROSALUD established the policy of signing a "letter of intention" with the authorities, in which it was agreed that PROSALUD would carry out market studies as a basis for defining the location of the planned clinic or clinics. This procedure put PRO-SALUD in the position of an investor that was not going to invest its resources in a place where the desired results could not be obtained. In practice, the negotiation of each clinic had particular features and the lessons learned from these experiences permitted PROSALUD to perfect its mechanisms for gaining the support of the authorities.

Designing the Clinics

The first PROSALUD clinics did not have a well-defined identity and physical characteristics, probably because no health care delivery model had been developed as the basis for their design. Because the organization's strategic vision was not well defined, the structure of clinics could not follow from it. For example, the first clinics were located in existing public-sector facilities. This did not work because PROSALUD adapted the clinics' function to the available structures rather than changing it.

With the evolution of a conceptual model came the definition of how services should operate and the necessity of adapting the structure of clinics to their function. New clinics had to be designed to be compatible with the service delivery model, and existing clinics had to be remodeled.

The next step was defining a model structure that would be compatible with the way in which services operated. Functional areas and minimum and maximum sizes for each area were developed as standards for physical plants. Initially for marketing reasons and later as part of the franchising system, standards were set for the appearance of clinics: colors and exterior and interior decoration were standardized.

Organizing Health Services

Integrating Preventive and Curative Services

Although the development of the package of services was largely based on the standards of the MOH, integrating the services posed a major operating problem. In principle, the staff fully accepted the concept of integration but in practice it was very difficult to accomplish because the majority of the personnel came from the MOH, where health services were not delivered in an integrated way.

The most significant problems were integrating services at the staff level and establishing schedules. The goal was for all clinic personnel to provide both preventive and curative services during regular working hours (without special hours). Many staff members resisted having to provide preventive and curative care. This obstacle was overcome by training staff and using medical records in which curative and preventive care were combined. As expected, the nursing staff accepted the new system better than did the doctors, who had more difficulty in adjusting to it.

This effort succeeded in increasing productivity by eliminating the need for staff dedicated to preventive care or family planning. It also made special schedules or days for preventive programs unnecessary. This was a major efficiency gain in labor costs.

Setting Prices

Prices required special attention, both in their establishment and their application. In setting prices, the major problem was the lack of internal cost parameters and of previous experience. The first fees were based on the fees charged for similar services in public-sector centers. PRO-SALUD established the principle that preventive services would be free of charge while curative services would be subject to fees.

In practice, the fee-for-service system made it more complex to set the prices of some services. For example, determining the price of maternity care was difficult because of the need to determine the cost of the services, drugs, and other products each patient received or used. And clients who for medical reasons required more services represented an excessive cost for such a system. For these reasons, PROSALUD changed the basic package of services in some cases. To continue with the example of maternity care: a single fee was set, and it included all the drugs received. The idea was that the same price would be charged for any service regardless of its actual cost. Thus, some services cost less than the price charged. The surplus revenue subsidized those patients for whom the price charged was less than the actual cost of services. An advantage of this pricing was that the client would know the total cost of the service in advance and not fear having to pay for "extras."

Another example was including follow-up visits for the same episode of illness in the fee charged for a medical consultation. Clients received the message that PROSALUD physicians offered them the opportunity to return to the clinic, at no additional cost, if their condition did not improve or if they needed follow-up care indicated by their physician. In this way the medical consultation became a package that included an initial consultation and follow-up for the same illness episode.

PROSALUD was able to determine the actual costs of services due to the development of the management information system and to use this information to support decision-making about prices with objective data. The development of the cost accounting system was important not only for determining the prices of services but also for adapting service packages and evaluating the capacity of the organization to implement cross-subsidies.

In applying prices, the first obstacle was to educate staff about the reasons for charging fees for services. Some staff members, especially those from the public sector, were not convinced that fees were necessary. This attitude had practical repercussions for the collection of fees. Thus the training of staff was oriented toward changing their perceptions about charging fees for services, so that they would see it as an essential component of the sustainability of the system.

Another issue was exemptions for the poor, as a means of increasing the equity of the system. The policy that was established initially allowed a degree of flexibility in who paid and who did not because there was no information about how people would react to the prices. The consequences of this policy were not positive, since there were abuses on the part of both clients and staff members. The idea of classifying clients by income was rejected because the cost of doing so was more than the incidental losses of fees caused by not limiting exemptions from fees sufficiently. The first measure taken to protect equity of access was establishing exemptions for indigent individuals, as determined by the head nurse (exemptions had previously been ill defined and were left up to the clinic receptionist) with input from the community health worker. PROSALUD later set maximum quotas that each clinic could use to subsidize the cost of care for the poor. When clinic staff became more involved in financial planning, they became more aware of the limits of the system and learned that it could afford to pay for only a portion of the care of low-income clients.

The idea of permanently categorizing a person or family as indigent was rejected, since it implied a permanent and automatic right to receive services. PROSALUD preferred to treat every case individually and apply exemptions or discounts as a special activity, based on the staff members' assessment of ability to pay and the urgency of the care needed. Despite efforts to limit exemptions to those who are most in need, the problem of balancing the need for fee revenues with equitable access to services has persisted.

Managing the Quality of Services

Although in principle all PROSALUD's managerial and operational staff agree about the necessity of providing high-quality services as one of the foundations of sustainability, in practice there are conceptual and operational problems that must be overcome.

Among the *conceptual* problems, the most significant was physicians' perception that users did not have the capacity to judge the technical quality of services. This perception corresponded to the "physician-centered model" of care, in which the doctors of the country have been trained and which made the doctor the sole judge of quality according to technical criteria. The opinions of users and criteria related to efficiency were not considered valid. This view was consistent with the traditional public-sector model, in which sustainability was not an issue. For PRO-SALUD it was essential to forge a new way of thinking because, among other reasons, the financial self-sufficiency of the system was based on the willingness to pay of the patient, who was, after all, the *client*.

Changing the view of the patient into that of the client was difficult because it implied putting the client at the center of the system, displacing the physician from her or his traditional role. Some doctors could not tolerate this change and had to leave the organization. Training and supervision played an important role in creating this new dimension of the organizational culture. As the organization matured, the quality of services came to be defined in a more integrated and comprehensive manner: technical or clinical quality, interpersonal quality, and managerial quality.

Among the *operational* problems, the most significant were related to the standardization of curative services and maternity services. The standardization of preventive services was simpler for two reasons: the existence of norms and protocols developed by the public sector, and the fact that the work is carried out by nurses and nurse's aides, who accepted the performance of standardized tasks more willingly. Standardizing curative services was particularly difficult because the doctors had been trained in different universities, where they learned different ways of treating cases, and they perceived standard treatment protocols as a threat to their freedom to choose the course to follow with each patient.

PROSALUD used training to change these practices, with disappointing results, given that there was no profound change in the way in which standard treatment protocols were followed. Participatory research (studies of knowledge, attitudes, and practices) on specific health conditions, such as the management of diarrhea in infants, acute respiratory infections, sexually transmitted diseases, and family planning, yielded better results.

Maternity care provides another example of problems in the application of protocols, which was made difficult by resistance based on prejudices or local customs. One of these customs was shaving the pubic area of women undergoing their first delivery, a practice that studies have shown is not only unnecessary but also increases the risk of postpartum infections and is uncomfortable for the woman. Doctors' resistance to change was minimized by using the medical literature and data from interviews with women who preferred more sensitive maternity care.

In addition to training and participatory research, clinic-level supervision played an important role in creating a culture of service quality centered on the client. In retrospect, this new focus also demonstrated that PROSALUD would not be sustainable without the development of a system of continuous quality improvement. Thus it was the point of departure in obtaining the commitment of clinic staff.

Human Resources Management Issues

Selecting and Hiring Staff

In Bolivia, the social problem of unemployment and the lack of systems for equal job opportunity mean that the unemployed generally seek employment through personal, family, or political influence. The result is that every job opening could become a source of discrimination, corruption, or violation of human rights. The most common problems that arise in hiring are

- lack of confidence on the part of those seeking employment in the process of selecting personnel, especially for publicly announced positions
- lack of systems and tools to ensure objectivity and transparency in the selection of personnel

- hiring decisions made by one person in an autocratic manner
- a view of work as a means of gaining power and the personal loyalty of those who attain a position.

At the beginning of the project, staff selection was not carried out in a systematic way. Although it was better than the public-sector system, it was still based on a mixture of technical criteria and personal preferences. The initial results were that the staff selected principally on the basis of technical criteria were more productive and more loyal to the organization. Staff chosen on the basis of more subjective criteria tended to be less productive and more loyal to the person or people who had helped them obtain a job. It became necessary to dismiss some inefficient employees as a result of these practices. These dismissals caused economic losses (because Bolivian law mandates the payment of three months' salary in the case of firing without criminal cause) and the intangible cost of a poor image of the organization.

Following these experiences, PROSALUD's management realized that staff selection in a system that aimed to be self-sustaining had to be performed in a systematic, objective, ethical, and transparent manner. The most important measures taken were (1) establishing a comprehensive selection system with standards and tools, (2) instituting mechanisms for decision-making that involved more than one person, and (3) informing all applicants for new jobs about this process and their right to appeal if they felt that there had been any irregularity in the process.

The enforcement of these measures, with complementary procedures (see the section of chapter 4 entitled "Human Resources Management"), permitted PROSALUD to establish an organizational culture of managing human resources in a technical but humane and transparent fashion. The major benefits of this approach were a high staff retention rate, a decrease in the number of dismissals, greater moral leadership on the part of management, and greater staff productivity.

When PROSALUD was replicated in other cities, staff selection was the first indicator for the authorities and local professionals that the organization was serious about doing business differently. Having an internal human resources policy and system permitted PROSALUD not only to contract with the personnel needed but also to manage and deflect pressures from some influential community members and government authorities.

Training Staff

At the start-up of PROSALUD, the rationale for unsystematic hiring practices might have been that good training could compensate for errors of selection. But in practice this was not the case, and it was necessary to incorporate training into staff selection. Staff training became the trial by fire of staff selection.

PROSALUD instituted a two-phase selection process. When vacancies occurred, it selected more candidates than it had positions for. Selection was preselection, in reality, because the potential appointees were required to undergo training not only in clinical or technical elements of the job but also in PROSALUD values, method of operations, and relations with patients and the community. This process inevitably resulted in a winnowing of the potential candidates for the vacancies. Either the candidates realized that they were not suited for the position or organization, or PROSALUD's assessment led to the same conclusion. For those candidates who successfully completed their training in the preselection phase, a second, more intensive training period was instituted. Candidates who reached this stage were still not assured of being confirmed for the vacancies for which they had applied, however. This more intensive training facilitated a further inculcation of PROSALUD values in staff and ensured that their clinical and technical skills were adequate for the task they were to perform. This process of training resulted in a more qualified and productive staff for PROSALUD.

The first training courses were basically technical and oriented toward maternal/child health programs. Management aspects were covered superficially, and theoretical topics were virtually nonexistent. As the project evolved conceptually, management issues became more important and they formed the central focus of the training. The challenge was to motivate clinical staff to evolve from a mentality of service delivery toward one of service management.

Once the "project" mentality changed to an "organizational" mentality, it became essential to incorporate theoretical and conceptual topics into training. The incorporation of staff into the organizational culture complemented the technical and managerial capacities that had already been developed.

In short, staff training evolved cumulatively from basically programmatic training to management training and finally to the transmission of PROSALUD's corporate culture. The desired outcome was a technically trained staff who had management skills and identified with the organization's philosophy.

Compensating Staff
One of the major problems in the public sector that PROSALUD had to face was offering an attractive compensation package that was competitive with the labor market but could at the same time be covered by the revenues from user fees. There were two basic problems in the public sector: low salaries and slow payment, both of which were tied to union activity. Delays in payment were easier to solve, and paying salaries punctually has become part of the organization's culture. In the Bolivian setting it is much appreciated by the staff.

In the first PROSALUD clinics, staff were paid solely on a salary basis. At that time salaries were approximately 50% higher than those in the public sector and therefore were highly attractive. This comparative advantage (the gap between public-sector salaries and those of PRO-SALUD) was gradually lost when the salaries became equal in 1995, but PROSALUD continued to have the advantage of prompt payment because delayed payment persisted in the public sector.

Staff compensation followed the same evolution as the conceptual model of PROSALUD. In the beginning (1985-86), the service delivery model was closer to the public-sector model, and it seemed logical that staff be paid on a salary basis. Beginning in 1987, the model incorporated specialists and dentists under fee-sharing arrangements. These professionals shared their fees with the system, while the medical director of the clinics and the rest of the staff received only salaries. The next step was the development of economic incentives based on productivity. This measure was revolutionary at that time. The outcomes were good, but the impact of the incentives on the staff diminished over time, and in 1998 they were discontinued due to new government regulations that obliged employers to include incentive payments in salaries.

To make up for this decrease in income, the general practitioners in the clinics, who were salaried, were authorized to work on Saturday mornings under a fee-sharing arrangement. The outcome was positive, and later the hours of emergency service were extended under the same arrangement so that these doctors could increase service delivery, their incomes, and clinics' revenues without incurring an increase in fixed costs.

As the gap between public-sector salaries and those offered by PRO-SALUD decreased, medical personnel put increasing pressure on the organization to pay higher salaries or raise the percentage of services for which PROSALUD split the fees with doctors. The percentage distribution of fees underwent some distortions because PROSALUD's portion did not grow at the same rate as its costs in some cases or take into account the difficulty of hiring doctors in clinics where prices were lower. Another problem was related to doctors' perceptions of differences in commissions for the same service (because the prices of services varied according to the clinic).

This problem has not yet been solved, although the proposed solution is to set the doctor's payment according to the service delivered, independent of the user fee. In this way the distortions produced by the payment system could be corrected. This system has many benefits but our experience with its application has revealed inequities that must be studied and rectified.

Negotiating with the Authorities

The processes and results of negotiating with the authorities varied widely and were successful to the extent that PROSALUD responded to their questions and concerns. One of the most difficult elements to manage was the perception of some authorities that PROSALUD was competing with the public sector and usurping a role that belonged exclusively to the government. For example, in the case of central-level MOH officials, one of the most significant problems was their desire to control the selection of staff. At the beginning of the project, the central MOH officials were more cooperative but as PROSALUD grew and its relative importance increased, the tensions became more obvious.

Relations with mayoralties were much more positive due to greater flexibility, especially after the Popular Participation Law was passed. Municipalities' acceptance of the PROSALUD model brought with it the advantage of new investments in health and the perception that local government was doing something for the community. However, there were difficulties, such as the desire of some officials to intervene in the selection of staff. Political conflicts between the MOH and the municipalities caused difficulties for PROSALUD and threatened the implementation of services. In fact, PROSALUD postponed its entry into a major city in Bolivia because the local MOH officials opposed, for political reasons, the city's initiative to introduce PROSALUD services.

Expansion Issues

The replication of the model in other cities of the country represented a great challenge simply because no one had experience in doing it and PROSALUD had to learn by doing. The MOH approved the idea of replicating the network in the cities of La Paz and El Alto, and USAID agreed to finance it through a cooperative agreement with PROSALUD. USAID provided long-term technical assistance through two members of the management team at headquarters and an expatriate technical advisor.

The major operational problems generally concerned the transmission of a corporate culture to a management and technical team that obviously had a very different way of seeing and doing things. The primary task turned out to be "selling" a new model, and the challenge was convincing the managers of the system of its viability so that they would internalize it. Some problems encountered and their causes were:

- The administrative manuals at headquarters had not been conceived with the idea of having a branch office or operations in other cities. As a result the manuals had to be adapted to the new situation.

- The management information system (MIS) was obsolete because it, too, had been developed without considering the possibility that offices and clinics might be established in other cities. To respond to this problem, PROSALUD contracted with a local firm to develop a new MIS that could handle future expansion.

- On one hand, applying the health care delivery model in the clinics was relatively easy. But this was not the case with the management model in the Regional Office of La Paz. The managers who were hired resisted the change, which caused problems in implementing the model. Their desire to change the model and do business in the usual way led to a lot of friction, which was overcome when everyone realized that the implementation process had to be flexible, without sacrificing the principles and basic characteristics of the model.

- On the other hand, the decision-making structure was complicated by the lack of tools for decentralized management of operations.

This need led to the formulation of policies and the refinement of technical and administrative manuals. The concept and methodology of franchising was important in enabling the decentralized management of the new networks that PROSALUD established.

- After La Paz and El Alto came the expansion of PROSALUD to other cities. The necessity of optimizing the use of management time led to the restructuring of the headquarters, by separating operational functions from management functions at the national level. In this way, PROSALUD decentralized the management of the clinics in Santa Cruz, and the National Office turned its attention to its role as "master franchiser" of the PROSALUD system in the country.

9
What Has PROSALUD Learned?

This chapter presents the most important lessons that PROSALUD has learned from its 14 years of experience. These lessons were learned from trial and error and are part of a continuing learning process with no blueprints. This chapter discusses some enabling factors; a central or other authority cannot, however, simply mandate them. Rather they must be recognized, carefully nurtured, and adapted to local situations if they are to be the building blocks of success.

Gaining Political Commitment

The impetus for change often arises from political pressures outside the health sector. Only rarely does the health sector itself spearhead efforts aimed at major restructuring of the health system. Even when it does, many central-level health managers actively resist the transfer of power. So when there is political commitment to solving health problems without being bound by past structures, there is the opportunity to introduce significant changes in how health services are organized and financed. For a radical model to succeed, key leaders must be committed to the concept and willing to see it through all the difficulties of implementation. Where such strong political support exists, the implementation of a private-public sector collaborative model is faster and more problem free. These leaders and those spearheading the innovative model being tested must be risk-takers. These individuals firmly believe in what is being tried and are willing to seek and apply innovative solutions to organizational and management problems. Such solutions may include allowing a degree of flexibility with rules and regulations that will facilitate the development of the model program, without compromising quality or the underlying principles.

Changes can occur when there are some guidelines about what is important. In Bolivia, the need for major changes came from the political sphere and enabled the "dreaming of big dreams" that in turn allowed the formation of PROSALUD. In proposing such changes, political leaders facilitated the development of the purpose, rationale, objectives, and implementation design, including a clear definition of roles for the various management levels and the linkages between them, of the PROSALUD model. A supportive government administrative head is thus a strong plus for setting up and running a decentralized public-private health or family planning program.

Using Market-Based Strategies

A fundamental understanding and application of basic market principles, such as supply and demand and the promotion of services, has been key to PROSALUD's activities. During the planning, establishment, and management of the organization's cost-recovery strategy, the analysis of market dynamics has consistently been utilized as a managerial tool. Using a market analysis approach in the decision-making process can include studies of the relationships among needs, supply and demand, as well as the market's relationship to morbidity and mortality trends ("felt needs" of consumers vs. "unfelt needs"); and the use of techniques that increase demand in health centers, while taking time and money constraints into account. These strategies increase the acceptability, accessibility, and affordability of the services offered.

Replicating the Model in Diverse Areas

The ability to replicate the PROSALUD model developed in Santa Cruz (located on a tropical plain) to areas that differ culturally, geographically, and economically has already been demonstrated in Bolivia. In 1991, the first replication exercise began in La Paz and El Alto cities (in the high mountains). Based on this experience, beginning in 1996 the model was expanded to Tarija (valley region), Yacuiba (Chaco region in the southeast), Riberalta (Amazonian region in the northwest), and

Puerto Quijarro (tropical region, east of Santa Cruz City). The greatest difficulty in assessing the success of replication is that it depends on so many different factors. Furthermore, the replication process accelerates the evolution of the model and affects the whole system, and its success is essentially based on people. Franchising methodologies and concepts were very useful tools in both the planning and the implementation phases. The model will continue to evolve as the organization strives to refine and improve to achieve increasing levels of coverage, quality, efficiency, and cost-effectiveness.

Replication Affects the Whole System

The replication process accelerates the evolution of the model and has an impact on the whole system. In other words, there are no static blueprints. As the model expands, each new center is carefully adapted according to the unique environment in which each operates. The lessons learned from these adaptations are valuable for adapting the overall model and they affect the next replications. One example of this is the evolution of the "basic clinic concept" to the "polyclinic concept" when PROSALUD was replicated in Tarija. This experience became the new trend in the network and a policy for future replications.

Franchising Is a Useful Tool

Franchising methodologies and concepts were very useful tools in both the planning and the implementation phases.

- In the planning phase, PROSALUD used a market demand and financial projection model as the basic tool to assess financial sustainability in a given area. The main inputs to this model came from a market study of needs and demand for services and an assessment of the supply of services currently available and their quality.

- In the implementation phase, PROSALUD relied on its operating manuals, protocols, procedures, and standards to foster a corporate culture in the new staff and ensure high quality of services.

The Success of Replication Depends on People

The replication process is based on people. Developing, implementing, and maintaining its management strategies and standards have depended in large part on the manner in which PROSALUD fosters motivation, commitment, and accountability in its staff. Thus selection and training of new staff are top priorities once a decision to replicate is made.

Creating a Network of Health Centers

To promote sustainability with a dramatically new model for organizing and financing health services requires the inclusion of several health centers, not simply a single facility functioning as a pilot or demonstration facility. This network is necessary because of the diversity of populations that are to be covered and the services offered. Some facilities and some services will have an easier time covering their costs, while others may have difficulty due to the population and economic characteristics of the catchment areas. By having a network of facilities, success does not depend on choosing a single area that has all the positive elements needed to allow it to succeed financially while providing needed and essential health services. This permits cross-subsidization of services between facilities and within a facility.

Subsidizing Services for the Poor

Enrollment of a cross-section of the community allows those who have the means to pay for their health services to help subsidize those who do not. The poor lack the ability to pay for all of their health services, which means that to meet their health care needs and to achieve financial sustainability simultaneously, there have to be enrollees who pay greater than actual costs and services priced higher than cost to subsidize the poor. Such practical elements of social solidarity are critical for success.

Building Capacity

Building capacity means increasing a person's or institution's ability to pursue a vision by successfully adapting to change. Capacity can take many forms: clinical skills, administrative skills, resources, knowledge, confidence, motivation, systems, experience, organizational learning, leadership, involvement of stakeholders, or quality improvement. PRO-SALUD found that the introduction of an innovative model greatly increased the need for skilled management. In many situations, qualified health managers with varied skills are in very short supply. Usually the existing management training capacity is inadequate to meet the rapidly growing needs of a new organizational structure.

For capacity building to succeed in a given context, a set of values that guide how it is approached and undertaken is needed. These guiding principles are essential, since capacity building is not a short-term activity. PROSALUD established a long-term commitment to developing its entire staff. It found that capacity building is a continuum and that staff members gradually increase their ability to manage a myriad of clinical, administrative, and managerial tasks.

Monitoring and evaluation must be conducted systematically and continuously and the resulting information used to improve services. The lack of monitoring and evaluation of the impact of decentralization is pervasive. When monitoring and evaluation occur, they are often an afterthought, once the process of decentralization has begun, and without any baseline data with which to compare later findings. Where local progress is closely monitored, a new "culture of accountability" can be observed.

Using an Endowment to Achieve Financial Sustainability

PROSALUD's endowment—a combination of seed capital from the US Agency for International Development, surplus operating funds, and interest income—is an essential component of achieving financial independence. This growing self-sufficiency has allowed PROSALUD to provide and continue to expand both the number and range of its health care services. The endowment will contribute to PROSALUD's becoming fully self-sustaining and maintaining prices that lower-income populations can afford.

Key Elements of Implementation

PROSALUD's experience suggests that the following elements are critical to the successful implementation of a sustainable primary health care network:

- public-private partnerships
- effective community outreach
- adequate donor funding and support, including appropriate technical assistance
- optimal utilization of financial resources
- comprehensive management information system
- provider incentives
- operations research
- high-quality services
- understanding market dynamics, resulting in careful distribution and location of health centers.

Forming Collaborative Relationships with Public-Sector Institutions

PROSALUD entered into many types of management agreements with public organizations. Some of the most notable collaborations were with the Office of the Mayor in Santa Cruz for the construction and operation of three semiurban health centers, and with the MOH to operate and manage several of their health clinics, including oversight of staff and compensation based on PROSALUD standards.

Developing Community Participation

An important factor in PROSALUD's experience is the degree to which the communities that the centers serve support them. Community participation was developed through agreements with local institutions, which varied with the community. Before beginning operations, PROSALUD negotiated an agreement with the community, formalizing their mutual support. Such agreements have been signed with local water cooperatives, health committees, and civic committees.

Building Capacity for Financial Management

Estimating demand and associated income and expenses is necessary and can be carried out only with a sound financial management system. Management Sciences for Health and PROSALUD developed a model for projecting demand for services by using patient utilization rates in conjunction with population census data collected in each area. It based costs on an economic model that took into account the estimated patient demand and the resources to be used at each center. PROSALUD also considered potential community support before making any final decision to move to a new location.

PROSALUD and MSH, with technical assistance from Stern & Co., developed a computerized, integrated financial management and service statistics package to help staff monitor financial and utilization data. These data increased the capability of managers to make projections for the coming year based on experience. Data on market size and share, patient utilization, service costs, and revenue are the essential variables for making annual financial forecasts.

Designing Provider Payment Incentive Systems

Provider payment incentive systems influence more than just costs. MSH and PROSALUD devised incentives to (1) encourage greater utilization of facilities and hence to reduce fixed overhead costs by tying a portion of the income of the providers and employees to the income of the health centers, and (2) share the financial risks and benefits of the operations among the employees. These were key elements to improving quality and increasing provider efficiency.

Using Operations Research

Even health delivery organizations need to conduct research. PROSALUD's managers made a conscious effort to test and evaluate different management and service delivery strategies. Operations research studies were carried out to determine the feasibility and impact of these strategies on the project and the possibilities for replication. Through these studies, it was possible to determine the factors that contributed to or detracted from program sustainability.

Emphasizing Quality Assurance

Quality assurance ultimately determines the acceptability of services to the public. Quality has always been one of the fundamental elements of

PROSALUD. It is particularly critical as clinics are trying to expand services and coverage. Without incremental improvements in quality, it is difficult to attract and retain the additional clients needed to reach financial sustainability and to manage the process of change.

Conditions Required for the PROSALUD Model to Succeed

It is essential to specify the main requirements for the PROSALUD model to succeed, to analyze whether the lessons learned can be applied in other countries:

- It requires a country setting where at least first-generation structural reforms are under way, and the environment is conducive to the development of the private sector.

There are macro-level conditions without which a system like PROSALUD cannot function. The model is incompatible with planned economies where the bases of a free market economy do not exist. Political stability and respect for private initiative are also required.

- It requires political support from health and local authorities and communities.

The development of the model requires strong political support initially. Without such support, it is not possible to establish the public-private partnership that is one of the bases of the model. Countries where the process of reforming the health sector is beginning can be very receptive to this type of initiative.

- It is more applicable in urban and periurban areas than in rural areas.

The model is better adapted to urban and periurban areas where there are larger populations with a greater ability to pay for services. In PROSALUD's experience, the model does not work well in areas of low population density.

- It depends on the availability of qualified human resources, especially a relative surplus of doctors.

It would be very difficult to make a system like PROSALUD function in areas where there is a scarcity of doctors. In such areas, doctors prefer to be salaried and would probably not accept working under a fee-sharing arrangement. This preference would result in very high fixed costs.

- It depends on the willingness and ability of the public sector to lease facilities.

One of the essential ingredients of the model is the provision by the public sector (MOH or municipalities) of facilities or land for the construction of clinics. If the public sector cannot or does not wish to furnish this infrastructure, a model of this kind simply cannot be implemented.

- It requires an initial seed capital investment.

Apart from in-kind contributions from the public sector, that is, physical facilities, it is essential to have start-up capital for operating costs and technical assistance. A project of this type requires seed capital and financial support to underwrite its development until it reaches self-sufficiency. In the case of PROSALUD, the support of USAID through 2002 will total $14 million, in the form of direct financial support, technical assistance, and the endowment.

- The population must be willing and able to pay for health services. Without continuing subsidies, the model is limited in its ability to cover the health care needs of indigent populations.

Health care for the poor is one of the areas in which the model is limited. The most that the current model can do is to provide free care to some indigent clients. The system of cross-subsidies has limits, in terms of the system's capacity to afford to provide services to people who have very little ability to pay. This constraint could diminish if the new Basic Health Insurance program (see the conclusion) operates as planned, which would give PROSALUD the opportunity to provide services to the poor and be reimbursed for them.

- There must be unmet health needs in the target population.

Sufficient demand for services must exist for the financial model to succeed.

- The model requires a critical mass of health centers to support its management.

A model of this type requires a high-performing management system. The cost of management can only be justified if its benefits are distributed in the greatest possible number of operating units. Experience has shown that attaining this critical mass is essential to maximize the sustainability of the system.

Conclusion

Major Challenges in PROSALUD's Future

PROSALUD has become one of the leading health care delivery models in Bolivia. Ironically, this achievement has become one of the obstacles to its self-sufficiency: it has spawned a number of competitive clinics using basically the same model. For this reason, PROSALUD recognizes that it cannot rest on its laurels but must continue to evolve and improve (Holley 1996). PROSALUD faces challenges that must be considered to predict how the organization will evolve in the years to come.

Achieving a Fully Autonomous Governance System

The USAID mission in Bolivia actively promoted the institutional autonomy of PROSALUD. The first evidence of its confidence in the organization was the establishment in 1991 of the cooperative agreement with PROSALUD for its replication in La Paz and El Alto. Subsequently, USAID provided direct grants that did not require substantial external involvement. Finally, in 1997, as an even greater proof of confidence, USAID approved the establishment of the endowment fund as part of a plan for financial sustainability. This action made it necessary to reform PROSALUD's bylaws and, as a result, to expand the Assembly of Associates and take other measures to advance the organization's development.

Since 1997 the Board of Directors has taken on more roles and responsibilities that, to some extent, have replaced those that USAID performed. The challenge is to consolidate this process to achieve a fully autonomous governance system. Thus the ultimate goal of this partnership will be realized: to ensure that the partner is able to continue long after the partnership is over.

Reaching Sustainability

Improving its financial position. Although the financial results achieved to date are encouraging, it is clear that the organization needs to accelerate processes that will improve its efficiency and its level of cost recovery to meet the deadline established in the long-term sustainability plan, of which the endowment fund is a part. The critical elements of this plan, which have already been put in place, include:

- increasing the demand for existing services
- accelerating the growth of new clinics
- broadening the types of services offered
- instituting measures to increase efficiency
- raising prices

Raising prices is the least attractive of these measures because it will not only impede the access to services of some people in the target population but also diminish demand. The achievement of the financial objectives depends to a large extent on maintaining the ability and willingness to pay of the target population. Given that the ability to pay is beyond PROSALUD's scope of influence, it must concentrate on providing the best value in the services delivered to generate the volume of demand needed to support this model.

Increasing the endowment fund. Another major challenge is to increase the endowment fund with contributions from other donors, thereby increasing the organization's capacity to respond to the needs of the target population. The stage of development that PROSALUD has reached in providing health services to underserved populations enables it to offer good "returns on investment" to potential donors to its endowment fund. It is likely to meet this challenge because PROSALUD has demonstrated its capacity to manage the organization and its endowment fund.

Leadership

Maintaining innovation and entrepreneurial vision. As organizations mature, they tend toward maintaining the status quo, putting at risk everything that they have achieved. One of the distinctive features of PROSALUD has been introducing a culture of innovation, both conceptual and operational. It will be essential to maintain this entrepreneurial vision to face external challenges.

Playing an active role in health sector reform. The process of reform in Bolivia's health sector is irreversible and is achieving considerable advances. The introduction of PROSALUD into the reform process in Bolivia is an opportunity and a very important challenge to strengthening and consolidating public-private partnerships.

When the Bolivian government launched the National Insurance for Mothers and Children program (Seguro Nacional de Maternidad y Niñez or SNMN) in mid-1996, its design excluded the possibility of participation by nongovernmental organizations. It was oriented instead toward increasing the utilization of public-sector services through the elimination of economic barriers by providing free care and subsidies. In practice, it involved the provision of 20 different health services incorporated into a minimum package that the whole population had the right to receive.

Because the National Insurance program was conceived as a public-sector effort, the conditions set for NGOs were very disadvantageous. PROSALUD did not join this program for economic reasons and because it lacked confidence in its continuity. On the economic side, the program paid only the variable costs of services and not the fixed costs (principally staff). This would have meant receiving only 40 percent of the total cost of services. In addition to very low salaries, there were administrative problems such as delays in payment and in the delivery of inputs (part of the subsidy was in-kind contributions).

If PROSALUD had joined this scheme, the economic consequences would have been disastrous. The decision not to join entailed stepping up its promotion of maternal/child health activities, since PROSALUD now had to compete with free services. For some MOH officials, this competition suggested that there would be a significant reduction in PROSALUD's services, which would eventually lead to its collapse. Overall, however, the number of maternity services decreased only 9 percent in the first year of the National Insurance program. The greatest decrease took place in the clinics of the city of Santa Cruz, while, paradoxically, in the clinics of El Alto, the poorest periurban zone in the country, the number of maternity services increased slightly.

The lessons for PROSALUD were that the apparent economic barrier did not play a great role and that quality of services was the way to retain clients. This was clearly a critical moment in the partnership of PROSALUD and the MOH, but, for the structural reasons discussed above, it was impossible for the NGO sector to participate in the National Insurance scheme.

In August 1997, the new government proposed the creation of Basic Health Insurance (Seguro Básico de Salud) to expand the reach of the National Insurance program (which covered only mothers and children). Launched at the beginning of 1999, the new insurance program created the conditions for true strategic alliances among multiple service providers, including NGOs. Its design was based on the principles of efficiency and competitiveness. New possibilities opened up for PROSALUD to be able to participate fully. In the Basic Health Insurance program, NGOs could not only provide services and be better compensated for them, they could also receive resources from government investments.

Although there are still many questions about how this initiative will be implemented, there is a great opportunity and challenge on the horizon for PROSALUD: to incorporate itself into the Basic Health Insurance program and thus consolidate the model of public-private partnerships for the benefit of the population it serves.

The Application of the PROSALUD Experience in Other Countries

The City+Med project in Haiti was the first project to apply components of the PROSALUD model, in a network of private clinics in Port-au-Prince. Some of the lessons learned and basic concepts of this model have been successfully applied since 1991.

The US Agency for International Development also considered PROSALUD to be a model of such potential that it initiated the development of a similar system in Peru in 1995 to demonstrate that the model is not limited by the cultural and social characteristics of Bolivia. The Maxsalud project in Peru has opened four clinics and received funding from USAID to add four more clinics. PROSALUD provided technical assistance in the design of this project.

From 1993 through 1998, Management Sciences for Health and PROSALUD provided technical assistance to APROFAM, the Guatemalan affiliate of the International Planned Parenthood Federation, to improve the sustainability of its network of urban clinics. Some of the lessons learned from the PROSALUD experience were applied, and positive results were observed in the sustainability of this organization.

In conjunction with the government of the Republic of Zambia's health reform initiative, the Ministry of Health asked Population Services International to carry out a feasibility study in 1995 to determine whether private-sector franchising techniques could be used to increase the delivery of primary health care services to lower- and middle-income Zambians. In 1996, the British Overseas Development Administration (now the Department for International Development) provided financial support to conduct the study. The study team reviewed the experiences of social franchising projects worldwide, identified PRO-SALUD in Bolivia, and researched the feasibility of adapting this model to the Zambian context. The study concluded that "franchising a network of institutionally and financially sustainable clinics in Zambia to provide high-volume, quality health care at low to moderate fee levels would be feasible and would increase the efficiency, coverage, and utilization of the country's overall primary health care delivery system" (Population Services International 1996, pp. 1–2).

In Nicaragua, the Commercial Market Strategies Project and PRO-FAMILIA will work together from 1999 to 2001 to implement the Franchised Clinic Network Project, with $5.5 million in funding from USAID. The objectives of the project are to increase opportunities and incentives for private providers to deliver essential health services and expand access to an affordable package of services through the private health sector. This new project will draw on PROSALUD's experience to create a franchised, largely self-financing network of six to eight private-sector clinics that will provide high-quality, low-cost, integrated services to approximately 240,000 lower- to middle-income Nicaraguans.

The Franchised Clinic Network Project is designed to complement, rather than compete with, the public and private health sectors. PRO-FAMILIA clinics will be strategically located in lower- to middle-income areas affected by Hurricane Mitch and currently underserved by the existing health care system. USAID funds will cover clinic construction, equipment, operating costs, management, and technical assistance. All preventive care and other services included in priority public health campaigns will be provided to clients free of charge. Revenues generated from fees for curative care will cover the bulk of the cost of providing all services. It is expected that the network will be capable of recovering a large portion of recurrent costs from user fees.

For those interested in improving sustainability as a means of providing health care for more people, all these experiences represent new opportunities for experimentation and refinement of ideas, including looking at variations of existing strategies and new solutions to respond to the specific conditions of a country or region.

References and Resources

Blaney, C. L. "Making Motherhood Safer in Bolivia." *Network* 14, No. 3 (1994): 18–19, 27.

Collins, James C., and Jerry I. Porras. "Building Your Company's Vision." *Harvard Business Review,* Sept.–Oct. 1996: pp. 65–77.

Family Planning Management Development Project. "Focusing on Customer Service." *Family Planning Manager* 5, No. 1 (1996): 1–18. Boston: Management Sciences for Health.

———. "Forming Partnerships to Improve Public Health." *The Manager* 7, No. 1 (1998–99): 1–26. Boston: Management Sciences for Health.

Fiedler, John L. "Organizational Development and Privatization: A Bolivian Success Story." *International Journal of Health Planning and Management* 5, No. 3 (1990): 167–86.

Fiedler, John L., and Lee R. Hougen. "Mid-Term Evaluation of the Self-Financing Primary Health Care II Project (PROSALUD) (511-0607)." POPTECH Report No. 95-034-029. Washington, DC: POPTECH for USAID/Bolivia, September 1995.

Fiedler, John L., Nancy Pielemeier, and Pamela Putney. "Final Evaluation: Bolivia Self-Financing Primary Health Care Project (511-0607)." Washington, DC: Management Systems International for USAID/Bolivia, 1989.

Hartman, A. Frederick. "Evaluation of the Impact of Health Services." Prepared for USAID/Bolivia. PROSALUD International Workshop. Boston, MA: Management Sciences for Health, August 1990.

Holden, Paul, and Sarath Rajapatirana. *Unshackling the Private Sector: A Latin American Story.* Directions in Development Series. Washington, DC: World Bank, 1995.

Holley, John. "Financial Projections and Strategy for PROSALUD." Partnerships for Health Reform Project. Bethesda, MD: Abt Associates, May 1996.

Huff-Rousselle, Maggie, and Catherine Overholt. "PROSALUD: Marketing and Financing Primary Health Care." Economic Development

Institute, The World Bank, *OGN Publications* 2 (1990): 1–18.

International Planned Parenthood Federation. "Country Profiles: Bolivia." http://www.ippf.org/regions/countries/bol/index.htm (Sept. 17, 1999).

Kapustin, Wendy. "PROSALUD: A Reengineering Model." Washington, DC: USAID, November 1996.

Martin, R. R., P. O'Connor, O. Wolowyna, and E. Duarte. "Evaluation of A.I.D. Child Survival Programs: Bolivia Case Study." AID Technical Report No. 5. Washington, DC: USAID, Nov. 1992.

Ministry of Health (MOH). "Plan Nacional de Salud Reproductiva y Supervivencia Infantil" (National Reproductive Health and Child Survival Plan). La Paz : MOH, 1989.

Newbrander, William, et al. *Guidelines for Achieving Equity: Ensuring Access of the Poor to Health Services under User Fee Systems.* Arlington, VA: BASICS, 1999.

Nogales, Javier. *La nueva política económica en Bolivia.* La Paz: Los Amigos del Libro, 1989.

Pan American Health Organization (PAHO). "Bolivia." In "Country Health Profiles." *Health in the Americas* (1998). http://www.paho.org/english/country/htm (July 6, 1999).

"Pildoras y preservativos al alcance de todos: En marcha Programa de Mercadeo Social." *Opciones* 1, No. 10 (1996).

Population Communication Services. "Final Report: Population Communication Services, the Johns Hopkins University, Project LA-BOL-04: Strategic Planning for Santa Cruz." Baltimore: Johns Hopkins School of Public Health, Center for Communication Programs, June 1994.

Population Services International (PSI). "Improving Health Care in Zambia through the Franchising of Private Sector Clinics." Washington, DC: PSI, December 1996.

PROSALUD. "Corporate Bylaws." Santa Cruz: PROSALUD National Office, 1997.

———. "Endowment Request to USAID." 1996.

———. "Health for Bolivia." Santa Cruz: PROSALUD National Office, 1999.

———. Home page. http://www.prosalud.org.

———. "Imagen corporativa." Santa Cruz: PROSALUD National Office, 1994.

———. "El libro azul de PROSALUD." Handbook for Employees. Santa Cruz: PROSALUD National Office, 1997.

————. "Manual de control de calidad." Santa Cruz: PROSALUD National Office, 1994.

————. "Manual de manejo de recursos humanos." Santa Cruz: PROSALUD National Office, 1996.

————. "Manual de organización y funciones." Santa Cruz: PROSALUD National Office, 1996.

————. "Manual de procedimientos técnicos y administrativos." Santa Cruz: PROSALUD National Office, 1996.

————. *PROSALUD para Bolivia: Annual Report 1997.* Santa Cruz: PROSALUD National Office, 1997.

————. *PROSALUD para Bolivia: Annual Report 1998.* Santa Cruz: PROSALUD National Office, 1998.

————. "Sistema de información gerencial." Santa Cruz: PROSALUD National Office, n.d.

Richardson, Paul, et al. "Quality, Costs and Cost Recovery: A Comparative Study of the Unidad Sanitaria of the Ministry of Health (MOH) and PROSALUD in Santa Cruz, Bolivia." Final Report for the MOH and USAID/Bolivia. Latin America Health and Nutrition Sustainability Project. Washington, DC: University Research Corporation and International Science and Technology Institute, September 1992.

Rosenthal, Gerald, Kevin Driessen, and Alfredo Solari. "Evaluation of the Primary Health Care Self-Financing Project (511-0569)." Washington, DC: USAID, 1986.

Rosenthal, Gerald, et al. *Toward Self-Financing of Primary Health Services: A Market Study of PROSALUD in Santa Cruz, Bolivia.* Health Care Financing in Latin America and the Caribbean Research Report No. 6. Stony Brook, NY: State University of New York at Stony Brook, 1988.

Sacca, Stephen. "A Step Closer to 'Health for All by the Year 2000'—A Critical Analysis of the Potential for Replicating a Self-Financing Primary Health Care Delivery System Based on the PROSALUD Experience in Bolivia." MA thesis. Cambridge, MA: Massachusetts Institute of Technology, 1990.

Straughan, Baird. "Self-Financing Health Project Brings Quality Care to Bolivia's Poor." *Front Lines.* Washington, DC: USAID, Feb. 1992.

United Nations (UN). "Basic Social Services for All." Wall chart. New York: UN Population Division, Dept. for Economic and Social Information and Policy Analysis, 1997.

United States Agency for International Development (USAID). "Bolivia

Country Health Profile." In "Latin America and the Caribbean: Resources." http://www.info.usaid.gov/countries/bo/bolipro.txt (Oct. 19, 1999).

———. "Self-Financing Primary Health Care." Project Paper, Project No. 511-0569. Washington, DC: USAID, 1983. (PNA-AAP-158)

———. "Self-Financing Primary Health Care." Project Paper, Project No. 511-0569. Amendment No. 1. Washington, DC: USAID, 1987. (PD-AAW-747)

———. "Self-Financing Primary Health Care." Project Paper, Project No. 511-0569. Amendment No. 2. Washington, DC: USAID, 1988. (PN-ABM-312)

Webb, Anna Kathryn Vandever, et al. *The Participation of Nongovernmental Organizations in Poverty Alleviation: A Case Study of the Honduras Social Investment Fund Project.* Washington, DC: The World Bank, 1995.

Index

About the Authors

Carlos J. Cuéllar has been the Technical Director of the Commercial Market Strategies Project (CMS) since January 1999. CMS is a USAID-funded project that aims to increase the involvement of the private and commercial sectors in health.

Dr. Cuéllar cofounded PROSALUD, of which he was the Executive Director until 1998, when he moved to the United States to work for Population Services International, one of the consortium members of CMS. He continues to serve PROSALUD as a member of the Assembly of Associates and a consultant.

Dr. Cuéllar has been providing technical assistance to improve health care institutions and programs in Latin America and the Caribbean and Africa for more than 12 years. His areas of expertise include public-private partnerships, private-sector networks, health services franchising, NGO sustainability, marketing of health services, and health financing. He worked for the Bolivian Ministry of Health for 5 years, first as an Epidemiologist in the National Tropical Diseases Center, then as a District Medical Officer in a rural area and, finally, as the Regional Health Officer of Santa Cruz.

He earned his MD from the Catholic University of Córdoba in Argentina, his MPH from the Institute of Tropical Medicine in Antwerp, Belgium, and a Diploma in Management and Administration from NUR University in Santa Cruz, Bolivia.

William Newbrander, the Director of MSH's Health Reform and Financing Program, is a health economist with 17 years of experience in health financing and hospital administration. He joined MSH in 1992 after having served with the World Health Organization for 8 years in Papua New Guinea, Thailand, and Switzerland. In addition to managing the MSH program, he provides technical assistance in health reform, national health insurance, hospital management, and decentralization.

Dr. Newbrander regularly teaches health financing at MSH, the Boston University School of Public Health, the World Bank, and other organizations. He recently directed an international team of experts who studied health sector reform in six Asian countries. That work was the focus of an Asian Development Bank regional conference on issues related to the growth of the private health sector.

His publications include a book based on the conference, *Private Health Sector Growth in Asia: Issues and Implications,* and a monograph on decentralization coauthored with Dr. Riitta-Liisa Kolehmainen-Aitken. He also coauthored *Modelling in Health Care Finance: A Compendium of Quantitative Techniques for Health Care Financing* and *Guidelines for Achieving Equity: Ensuring Access of the Poor to Health Services under User Fee Systems.* He holds master's degrees in Hospital Administration and in Economics as well as a PhD in Health Economics from the University of Michigan.

Gail Price, a Senior Program Associate in MSH's Population and Reproductive Health Program, manages MSH's domestic activities. Ms. Price has spent much of her career identifying ways in which health care systems in different countries can learn from each other. At MSH, she was the Project Director for Community Health Centers around the World: An International Exchange, a partnership between MSH and the National Association for Community Health Centers. She also worked with community health agencies as Coordinator of the Massachusetts Lessons without Borders program, a USAID initiative to bring the lessons of international development to the United States.

Ms. Price previously worked for the Boston Department of Health and Hospitals, where she was instrumental in launching Healthy Boston, a citywide initiative through which community coalitions assessed local needs and implemented projects to meet them. She completed her master's degree at the Harvard School of Public Health.

About Management Sciences for Health

Management Sciences for Health, Inc. (MSH), is a private, nonprofit organization, dedicated to closing the gap between what is known about public health problems and what is done to solve them. Since 1971, MSH has collaborated with health decision-makers throughout the world to improve the quality, availability, and affordability of health and population services.

MSH has assisted public and private health and population programs in over 100 countries by providing technical assistance, conducting training, carrying out applied research, and developing systems for health program management. MSH maintains a staff of more than 400 in its Boston, Massachusetts headquarters, offices in Washington, DC, and field offices throughout the world.

We provide long- and short-term technical assistance in six areas of expertise:

- health reform and financing
- primary health care and maternal/child health
- population and reproductive health
- information for management
- management training
- drug management

Recent and ongoing major efforts by MSH to address problems in public health include the following:

- MSH currently manages two multinational projects funded by the US Agency for International Development (Family Planning Management Development and Rational Pharmaceutical Management).

- MSH is also carrying out several national projects, including three in Africa (Guinea, Kenya, and South Africa), one in Haiti, one in Nicaragua, and one in the Philippines.

- We recently concluded successful work on the Madagascar APPROPOP/Family Planning and Senegal Child Survival and Family Planning projects.

- MSH is the managing partner of the Partnership for Child Health Care, Inc., which implements USAID's flagship child survival project, Basic Support for Institutionalizing Child Survival (BASICS).

- We have also been awarded a contract to carry out global technical assistance under the Maternal Child Health Technical Assistance (TASC) activity.